BUFF
Brides

BUFF
Brides

The Complete Guide to Getting in Shape

and Looking Great for Your Wedding Day

Sue Fleming

VILLARD NEW YORK

LIBRARY OF CONGRESS CATALOGING-IN-PUBLICATION DATA
Fleming, Sue
Buff brides : the complete guide to getting in shape and looking great for
your wedding day / Sue Fleming.
p.   cm.
Includes index.
ISBN 0-375-75855-0
1. Physical fitness for women.   2. Brides—Health and hygiene.   I. Title.
GV482 .F59 2002
646.7'5—dc21   2001049245

Villard Books website address: www.villard.com

Printed in the United States of America on acid-free paper

6   8   9   7

Book design by Jessica Shatan

To my wonderfully supportive friends and family

Contents

Introduction

QUOTES FROM THE BATTLEFIELD

*"The photographer will be taking pictures from
every angle and I do not want to get
back shots with the 'waving wattle'!"*

"I must have toned arms, I'm wearing a sleeveless gown!"

*"This is the most important day of my life.
I'll do whatever it takes to get in shape!"*

As a certified personal trainer who has worked in the health profession for more than ten years, I constantly hear concerns like these from nervous brides-to-be. Over time, I began to notice that more than half my clients were panicked women who gave me six months' notice to get them into "gown shape," so it seemed only natural to develop a fitness guide that would be useful for such a large population. The majority of my clients are women looking for custom-made weight training and fitness programs to prepare them for their wedding day—the day they consider the most important of their lives. Brides-to-be have the mentality "This time I'm going to do it!" and it gives me great pleasure to see them accomplish their goal. My clients are aware that wedding cake and flowers make a great impression; however, those things are gone before the next day. Photographs last forever!

Every year, 2.4 million women in America get married. Each bride starts planning her wedding with a vision of what she wants her special day to be like. I have spent countless hours with panicked brides-to-be who are united by the same goal: to look great and be in shape on their wedding day. Every little girl grows up with the vision of walking down the aisle in her beautiful gown. We've all dreamt about what that gown will look like, how perfect we will look, how wonderful we will feel. Why not make that dream a reality? The exercises outlined in this book will make that dream come true!

A wedding is a milestone in your life. There are three major rites of passage in most people's lives: birth, marriage, and death. This is the only one over which you have complete control—so take advantage of the fact! This book is your personal guide to looking and feeling your best for your big day.

Over the past few years, weddings have changed drastically. There are many new trends and ideas when it comes to the ceremony and reception. This holds true for bridal fashions as well. Today's wedding gowns are sleeker—many styles are cut low and show off the body. This is a huge concern for many of my clients, each of whom has a "problem area" that makes her feel self-conscious.

That is exactly what makes *Buff Brides* an essential tool for all brides-to-be. It integrates strength training with cardiovascular fitness training for optimum results. This book will guide you through the most effective exercises targeted to brides' most troublesome areas. Just like planning a wedding, working out is a commitment. I tell all my brides-to-be that in order to see results you have to be consistent. The workouts in *Buff Brides* are practical, easy to follow, and successful. There are no short-cuts, however; you have to make the commitment.

You may be asking yourself, "Does the *Buff Brides* workout guide really work?" Yes, it does, and I have the success stories to prove it, from people who didn't give up. Perhaps at times they lost some of their drive for fitness, but they kept up their commitment to the program anyway. These brides-to-be found the exercises easy to do at home and fun; most of all, they obtained results! I want to share a couple of examples of clients who successfully made the *Buff Brides* commitment.

Elizabeth never had a problem with her weight. At 6 feet, 1 inch, she was tall, beautiful, and excited about her upcoming May wedding. One December morning, exactly five months in advance of the big day, her wedding dress arrived. As Elizabeth put on the dress for the first time, to her utter dismay it was too tight in the waist. Although she was tall and lean, her abdominals were her "problem area." The dress was fitted (like a corset) around the waist, so there wasn't much room to play with. When the shop owner was questioned, her response was "Oh, I know why that size doesn't quite fit. The dress you tried on was off the rack and had been stretched a bit by different-sized girls. We probably should have ordered you a size larger—but I know you'll fit into it in May." Upon further investigation of the dress by the seamstress, Elizabeth learned that only one inch (half an inch on each side) could be saved. She was in big trouble. She immediately phoned me and said, "Oh, my God . . . you know, I can't lose my waist. I'll have to have a rib removed like Cher!"

That's where it began. Elizabeth was a machine. We worked

out four times a week, utilizing the exercises outlined in this book. During her next two fittings she found her waist size was slowly coming around. The fourth and final fitting was four days before the big day itself. I accompanied Elizabeth to this monumental event. As she pulled the white wonder over her head and zipped it up—*it was too big!* Elizabeth had lost more than 13 pounds! The seamstress screamed, "Good girl! I'm so proud of you!" Her mom, who was also there, was relieved as well. In the end, the seamstress had to take in about two inches.

That's just one example of a panicked bride-to-be who found success through this program. You get the idea. Fitting into her wedding dress comfortably and looking her best is on the mind of every bride.

Here's another success story.

I received a panicked e-mail from Alison one chilly January morning. "Help! I'm getting married in June, and I must start working out tonight! I have only six months to get my arms ready for this wedding!" Fortunately, my schedule was clear that evening and I had the pleasure of meeting another future "success story."

What I found remarkable about Alison was her commitment to her goal: preparing her body to look its best on her wedding day. Her dedication was endless. Even a long day at work never caused her to cancel. She started working with me twice a week, then quickly added another session at six in the morning. She was tireless. We gradually began to see arm definition, flatter abdominal muscles, and stronger legs. With each challenge I presented to Alison, her response was "How many days until the wedding?" People began to notice her changed appearance; heads started to turn, and she was constantly asked, "Are you working out?"

Needless to say, Alison looked terrific on her wedding day. Her spaghetti-strapped gown looked fabulous with her toned biceps and triceps. Her posture was elegant as she walked down the aisle because of the various back-strengthening exercises we had done over the previous six months. But most of all, she felt healthy and happy, and she was proud of her accomplishments. Working out consistently also helped alleviate some of the stress that inevitably accompanies wedding-day preparations. And her dress fit perfectly. She knew that all of the hard work she had done during the past six months had been worth it.

Brides-to-be come in all shapes and sizes. No matter how thin they are, fitting into their wedding dress "just right" is still a big concern. "Cut," toned muscles have become a bridal obsession.

This book is for the everyday bride. In an ideal world, every woman planning to tie the knot could hire a personal trainer to help her prepare for her wedding day. However, a personal trainer is a luxury very few women can afford. Using my personal experience, I have developed a comprehensive six-month program as well as a three-month modified program (for the bride who's short on time). Both have proven to be successful with my clients. Conveniently, they can be done in your own home with minimal equipment.

Many of the brides-to-be I train have similar questions and concerns with regard to fitness. Here are just a few of the most commonly asked questions.

Can I change my figure with a fitness program?

You can't change what God gave you—your body frame is yours to keep. But you *can* improve and sculpt what you have. You do have the ability to lose body fat and increase the amount of lean muscle in your body.

If I do 200 crunches a day, will I have flat abs?

This has to be the most frequently asked question I encounter. Women look in the mirror and want to focus in on their "problem" areas, such as abs, saddlebags, or flabby arms. Focusing on just one body part, or "spot reduction," doesn't work. You have to work on the whole package. In order to reduce any part of your body, you need to incorporate proper diet and exercise into your daily routine. As you work on your body as a whole, the unwanted problem areas will slowly cease to exist.

Can you recommend a good diet?

I think "diet" is a bad word. It implies starving yourself. Most "diets" are unbalanced; they do more harm than good. Some of the trendy diets on the market today lead to bad eating patterns that continue throughout life. My advice is to start by making small changes in your eating habits. Add new vegetables to your diet, cut out "hidden fats" like the ones found in salad dressings, drink more water (eight to nine glasses a day), and strive for balance. Your diet should contain a healthy balance of protein (15 to 20 percent), fat (less than 30 percent), and carbohydrates (50 to 55 percent). The only way to eat well and lose weight is to incorporate healthy eating habits into your life. Don't sabotage your metabolism by starving yourself.

When strength training, which should I increase— weight or repetitions?

Muscles adapt very quickly to each challenge placed on them. Women think that they will "bulk up" if they add more weight to their strength training program. This is a common myth that I'm constantly fighting. It is nearly impossible for women to become bulky, as they simply don't produce enough testosterone.

The rule of thumb when strength training is that to add size to a given body part you should increase the weight and lower the number of repetitions. Decreasing the weight and increasing the repetitions tones and strengthens muscles. Increasing the number of sets uses more calories, thus burning more fat.

Will strength training make me sore?

You have to expect to have some soreness after the first few workouts, especially if you're a beginner. But you shouldn't feel as if you've been run over by a truck! If you find yourself sore after each workout, you're working too hard. Lower the amount of weight you are using until your body adjusts. It is also important to stretch before and after each workout to help alleviate muscle soreness.

If I stop exercising, will the muscle I gained turn into fat?

Muscles cannot turn into fat, but they can shrink when you stop exercising. Your body will not burn as many calories, and naturally, if you continue to consume the same amount of food, it will begin to store fat. Our body-fat reserves are huge. Muscles give the appearance of a leaner, sleeker body. Keeping them toned and conditioned will ward off your body's tendency to store fat.

How long should I rest between exercises?

If you're trying to burn fat, keep your heart rate elevated by incorporating shorter resting periods—30 to 45 seconds between sets. Generally, 30 to 60 seconds between sets is recommended. Larger muscle groups may need a little longer to recover. Never work the same muscle group two days in a row, as muscles need time to recover and heal.

As a health and physical education teacher and personal trainer since 1989, I am passionate about one thing: teaching people how to feel better. Encouraging people to incorporate new health habits into their lives is a priority with me. Making it fun is also important, not only with children but with adults as well. Through my teaching experiences, I have learned what most people want. Quick fixes are not the answer. A balanced, sensible health and fitness program is. We live in a society where our children are exercising less, fast foods are a daily convenience, and eating disorders are abundant. As a physical education teacher, I have seen what these bad habits are doing to our children and teenagers.

If you are a bride-to-be, you have a lot going on as you prepare for your wedding. Don't think of this guide as a "quick fix." It will "reshape" your life as it directs you toward a healthier lifestyle.

So jump in and start today! Start believing, and incorporate a healthy fitness program that really works into your life. Each and every exercise and fitness tip in this book has proven successful with my clients—and not only for the wedding day. Most of my clients continue with the *Buff Brides* program and experience continued success, even after the wedding gown has been put away. The women who have continued with the programs in this book have learned to eat better, exercise regularly, and, most of all, feel better.

So throw away those bad habits, and let's get going! You're on your way to becoming a Buff Bride!

PART I

Getting Started

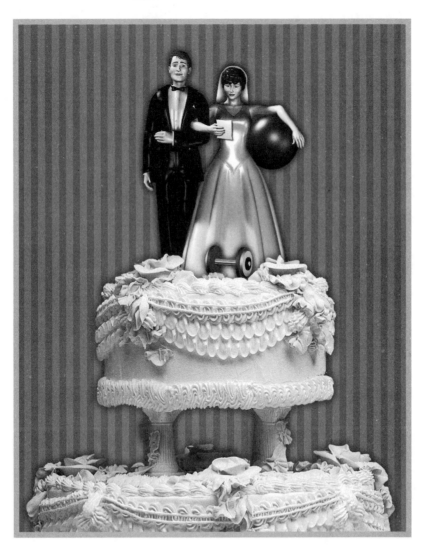

MOTIVATING YOURSELF

First and foremost, before you start any exercise program, you need to have had a physical and a clean bill of health within the last year. Once you get the OK from your doctor, you should be ready to start a gradual exercise program.

The hardest part about exercising is getting started. Everyone has a hundred excuses not to work out, including brides-to-be—and I've heard them all! Preparing for your wedding is time-consuming, but don't make that an excuse for not exercising. The time to start exercising was yesterday, but I'm willing to give you a break. The time to start is *now,* today, not next Monday! Don't think, "I'll do it later," because later *never* happens! *Suck it up,* put on your workout clothes, and get going! I tell my clients, "If it were easy, everybody would be doing it." Exercise is not easy; it's a commitment—just like planning a wedding. You wouldn't shortchange yourself on the cake and flowers, so why even think about shortchanging your own body? I always remind brides-to-be that the cake and flowers are forgotten after the wedding is over. But how many people leave their wedding picture on the mantel for the rest of their lives? If anything, that should be motivation enough! Who wants to look at her wedding picture year after year and regret not being in shape or even not feeling her best?

That's the beauty of this book. It focuses on simple, effective workouts that can be done in your own home. Most of the workouts outlined in the following pages can be completed, start to finish, in only an hour. That's all it takes! If you can, find a friend, a bridesmaid, your maid of honor—anyone who is willing to work out with you and motivate you—and do the program together. Brides often ask me, "When is the best time of day to work out?" There's a simple answer: The best time to work out is any time when you will actually do it. Try to schedule your workouts during the most convenient time of the day. If you have a busy schedule (as most of us do!), you must create the time. This book is not magic; you must make the commitment to work out consistently. Consistency yields positive results. I recommend working out at least three times a week; irregular training will take much more time to achieve results.

Most of all, make your training sessions *fun!* Wear exercise clothing that makes you feel good, even if you are training in the privacy of your own home. Put away the bulky leg warmers you haven't worn since 1987 and break out the sports bra! Reinforce feeling well by wearing something that makes you feel good!

The average American watches 12 to 15 hours of TV a week. Do you think on your wedding day you'll regret having missed another *Friends* rerun? Or will you wish you'd taken the time to get your arms looking like Jennifer Aniston's?

Incorporating exercise into your daily life should be a priority, whether you are getting married or not. Exercise affects your mood and will also increase your energy level. Again, schedule exercise into your day at a time when it's convenient for you, but don't procrastinate!

THE BEGINNING

Don't bite off more than you can chew. Most brides-to-be who start working out get frustrated early on because they try to do too much at the start. If the day after exercising you are so sore and achy that you can hardly move, you started at a level you weren't prepared for physically. More is not better when it comes to starting an exercise program. Feel good about your workouts, and don't expect your body to do something it can't.

The exercises described in Part II are designed to be done at home and in a limited workout space. I find that most of my clients lose motivation if they try to go to a public gym. Most of them have trouble just getting out the door! A simple workout that could be done in an hour becomes a two-hour ordeal. Getting to the gym, parking, and waiting in line to use the equipment can be frustrating and time-consuming! Most people don't have a lot of time to waste, and that is why the Buff Brides workouts are effective; they are simple and quick, and people stick with them!

With minimal equipment, you can sculpt, tone, and strengthen every major muscle group to improve the body areas emphasized by the type of wedding gown you have chosen. This book is geared to the bride-to-be who wants to save time, see results, and feel comfortable in her own home. Although this book focuses on strength training, I have also outlined some cardiovascular exercises that are crucial for a balanced workout. Stretching is another important part of your routine and should be done regularly to maintain and improve flexibility.

CREATING A HOME GYM:
SIMPLE ITEMS YOU WILL NEED TO BEGIN
YOUR STRENGTHENING PROGRAM

Creating a home gym can be very inexpensive. Of course, there are hundreds of expensive gadgets you can purchase. However, I am recommending what I feel is useful and will get the job done. You don't have to spend a lot of money to get into "bridal shape." Save the energy you'd spend on shopping for equipment and channel it into feeling good about your workouts and the positive results they will yield.

Dumbbells

Dumbbells come in various shapes, sizes, and colors. They also come in various prices. Think about it: a set of 3-pound dumbbells that costs $12 weighs the same as a set of 3-pound dumbbells that costs $25! Don't be fooled by fancy labels or advertisements. If you feel you'll be more inclined to use the more expensive dumbbells, go for them. But the cheaper models will do just as well.

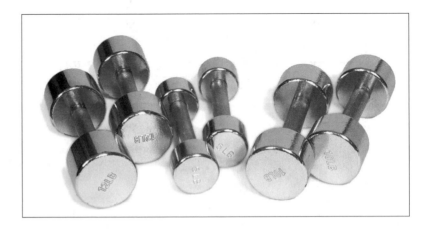

Depending on your level of strength, start off with three to four sets of dumbbells, increasing in weight. Beginners should start off with 3-, 5-, and 10-pound dumbbells. Intermediate and more advanced brides-to-be should start off with heavier weights: 5-, 10-, and 12- or 15-pound dumbbells.

I am an advocate of free weights because you can't "cheat" as much as you can when using machines. Let me explain: machines make things easier for you, as they direct your movement patterns. Free weights allow you to train each muscle group separately; your dominant side can't do all the work. Sometimes while you are using a machine, your dominant or stronger side will compensate for your weaker side when you start to get tired.

An Exercise Ball

An exercise ball is an excellent addition to your home gym. Traditionally, exercise balls were used by rehabilitation and physical therapy patients. Today they can be found in almost every gym. An exercise ball strengthens your core muscle group, the abdominal muscles and muscles of the lower back. These important muscles stabilize your body. Think of your body as a wheel. Your core is the hub of the wheel; your arms and legs are the spokes. If

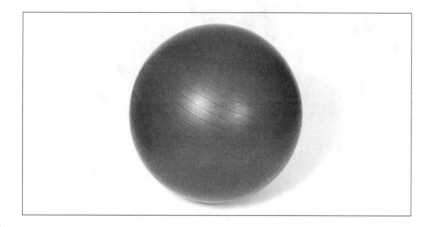

your core is weak, it will be difficult to strengthen other parts of your body. Often, people arch their back or release their abdominals when performing an exercise. This is usually a result of weak core strength. Many people compensate for this lack of strength by using their hip flexor muscles when performing abdominal exercises. The exercise ball strengthens the abdominals through a full range of motion without using the hip flexor muscles.

Core strength is important in developing and improving overall muscular strength. The exercise ball is especially useful for people with lower back pain because the ball supports the back muscles during the exercises.

An exercise ball usually comes with a pump. This allows you to inflate and deflate it quickly for easy storage. An exercise ball can also be used in place of a weight bench, which is especially useful for small apartments or workout areas. I recommend a 65-centimeter ball for the exercises in this book.

Step

I highly recommend purchasing a step for your home gym. Steps are inexpensive and provide a good cardiovascular work-

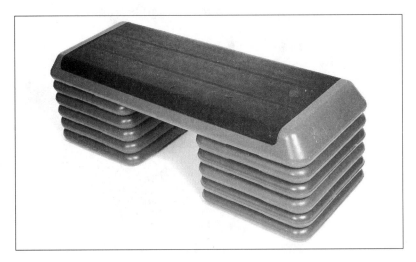

out as well as defining and toning the muscle groups of the lower body. Their lengths vary; I recommend anything from 28 inches to 43 inches. Lower lengths are great for small spaces.

Ankle Weights

Ankle weights can intensify your workout. They are worn around the ankle, usually attached by Velcro or clips. Some ankle weights have cylindrical weights that can be removed or added. I recommend these; as you get stronger, you will be able to adapt and not get stuck with a pair of weights you can't use. Ankle weights are relatively inexpensive, about $15 to $35.

An Exercise Mat

Unless your exercise space is carpeted, an exercise mat is a must, especially for a space with a hard floor. An exercise mat gives you the needed cushion for many of the stretches and strength training exercises outlined in this book. Mats are easy to store and are cheap, about $10.

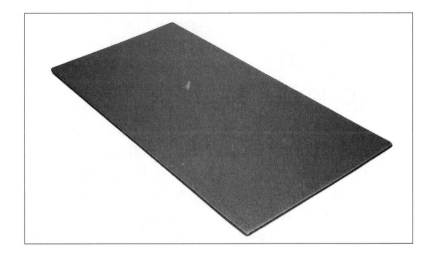

Weight Bench

Many of the exercises outlined in this book can be done with an exercise ball. However, if you have the space and money, a weight bench can be a good addition to your home gym. While a ball allows you to strengthen your core as well as other muscle groups, a bench will add variety to your workout. You could spend months picking out a bench, as they vary in size and price. Keep it simple! A good, sturdy bench can be purchased for $60 to $75. Some sporting goods stores offer a package deal if you purchase both dumbbells and a bench.

Shop around; a used bench can shave dollars off the price and be just as good as a new one! Many people sell their old ones, so look in your local newspaper classified ads. You might also try a used–gym equipment store. Make sure that the legs are stable and the padding is in good shape.

STRETCHING

Stretching is an integral piece of the getting-into-shape puzzle. Stretching improves your range of motion, and flexible muscles are less prone to suffering from soreness and injury. Increased flexibility enables you to get through everyday life much more easily. Well-stretched muscles appear leaner, and your posture improves. (Good posture should be on every bride's mind as she walks down the wedding aisle.)

Your body should be warm before you stretch. Try stretching a rubber band after it's been in the freezer all night! Your muscles need to wake up and warm up. A common mistake is jumping out of bed and starting a stretching routine. I recommend warming up for about 5 to 10 minutes before stretching. A warm-up can be very simple: jumping rope, running in place, or doing jumping jacks.

Stretching should be pain-free. Stretch to the point of mild discomfort or gentle tension, and don't forget to breathe! Your breathing should be slow, rhythmic, and under control. If you are bending forward on a stretch, exhale. Don't hold your breath while stretching. Also, keep your stretches slow and steady. Don't bounce! With a regular stretching routine, you will be able to reach and bend progressively farther.

Finally, stretching after a workout is just as important as stretching beforehand. When you're done with your exercise routine, cool down and stretch! Make sure to stretch the muscles that were utilized in your workout.

Simple, Effective Stretches

QUADRICEPS STRETCHES

Stand up straight with one hand on a support in front of you. Bend one leg back, holding the top of your foot. Keeping your knees together, bring your heel to your butt. Hold for 12 to 15 seconds, then repeat with the other leg. Do each leg twice.

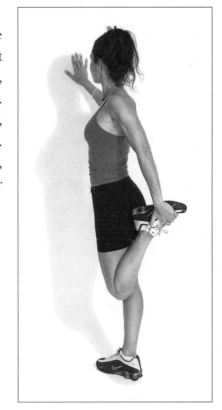

HAMSTRING STRETCHES

Lie flat on your back on an exercise mat or carpeted floor. Lift your left leg up perpendicular to the floor. Your right leg should be flat on the floor. Interlock your hands behind your left knee, pulling your leg toward your chest. Pull to where you feel a stretch in your left hamstring. Hold for 15 seconds then repeat with the opposite leg.

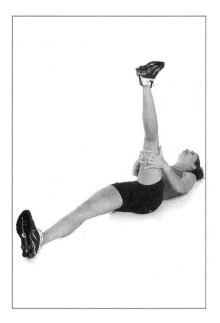

CALF STRETCHES

Standing, lean forward and place both hands on a wall or support in front of you. Keep one leg slightly bent and step back with the other leg, pushing your heel to the ground. Try to keep your heel down in order to bene-fit from this stretch. Hold for 12 to 15 seconds, then repeat. Do each calf twice.

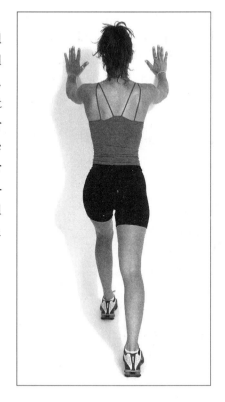

BUTT STRETCHES

Lie on your back with both feet flat on the floor. Cross your left leg over your right, above the knee. Grab your right leg behind your thigh (hamstring area) and pull both legs toward you until you feel the stretch in the left side of your butt. Hold for 20 seconds, then cross your legs the other way and stretch.

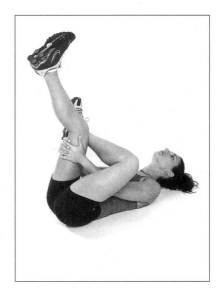

LOWER BACK/HIP/ HAMSTRING STRETCHES

Start in a standing position, feet shoulder width apart. Your feet should be pointed forward. Keeping your knees slightly bent, slowly bend forward from the hips. Let your arms and neck relax. Go to the point where you feel a slight stretch and hold for 12 to 15 seconds. To the count of four, return to the starting position. Repeat.

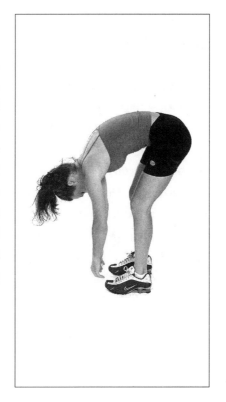

CHEST/SHOULDER STRETCHES

Standing, place your feet shoulder width apart. Don't lock your knees. Clasp your hands behind your back and lift your arms behind you. Keep your back straight. Hold for 12 to 15 seconds and repeat.

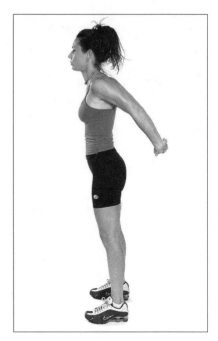

TRICEPS STRETCHES

Standing, place your arms overhead and hold the elbow of one arm with the hand of the other arm. Gently pull the elbow behind your head, feeling a stretch in the triceps. Breathe slowly, holding for 15 seconds. Switch arms and repeat. Do each arm twice.

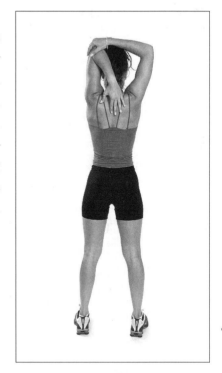

SHOULDERS/MIDDLE OF UPPER BACK STRETCHES

Standing without locking your knees, gently pull your elbow across your chest toward your opposite shoulder. Hold for 15 seconds, then repeat with the other elbow. Do each side twice.

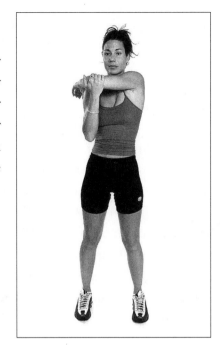

GROIN STRETCHES

Sitting on the floor, place your feet together so your heels are facing each other. Grab your ankles with your hands and lean forward slowly. Breathe slowly, holding the stretch for 15 seconds. Relax and then repeat.

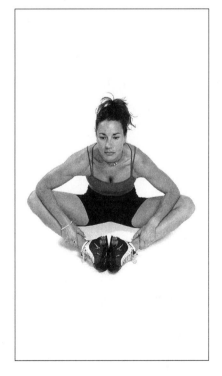

Measuring the number of times your heart beats per minute ensures that you are exercising at the right pace. Your heart rate (or pulse) can be taken very easily on the body, at either the wrist or the neck.

When exercising, you should aim to increase the number of times your heart beats per minute. This is called your target heart rate (THR). Your THR zone is 50 to 85 percent of your maximum heart rate (MHR), or the maximum number of times your heart can beat in one minute. Beginners should stay on the lower end of their THR to lower their risk of injury. When your level of fitness improves, exercise in the middle or upper end of your THR.

Here is a simple formula for determining your MHR:

$$220 - \text{age} = \text{MHR}$$

You can then figure your THR by calculating 50 percent and 85 percent of your MHR.

For example, for a 26-year-old woman:

$$\text{MHR: } 220 - 26 = 194$$

$$\text{THR } (50\%): 194 \times .50 = 97$$

$$\text{THR } (85\%): 194 \times .85 = 164.9$$

If your heart is beating below your 50 percent THR, you're probably not working hard enough. Push yourself a bit more.

If your heart is beating above your 85 percent THR, you're working too hard. Slow down or lower the intensity of the exercise.

BUFF *Brides*

Heart rate monitors worn on the body while exercising can help you monitor your THR. They can be purchased at any sporting goods store. You can also check your heart rate manually. Periodically during your workout, place your index and middle fingers in the groove on the side of your throat. Starting at zero, count how many times your heart beats in six seconds. Add a zero to that number. This is how many times (approximately) your heart is beating in one minute.

Monitoring your heart rate during exercise helps you push yourself. It can also warn you if you are working too hard.

Keeping track of your heart rate during the six-month and three-month *Buff Brides* workout programs will help you determine if your cardiovascular fitness is improving. Monitoring your heart rate after exercise is also important. The better shape you're in, the faster your heart rate will drop one minute after completing a cardiovascular exercise session.

HOW TO INTEGRATE CARDIOVASCULAR EXERCISE INTO YOUR WORKOUT

An effective workout is a *balanced* workout! Doing the same thing every day will not prepare your body for that special day. Stretching, cardiovascular activities, and strength training are the three elements of fitness training that will yield positive results. Most of my clients dislike incorporating cardiovascular activities into their workouts. One reason is "I don't have the time." Another, to put it bluntly, is "I hate it!" The key to successful cardiovascular training is to pick an activity you don't hate to do. Don't set yourself up for failure. Find something you like to do, and you'll be more likely to stick to it. In the next section, I will outline a few of the most popular, easier ways to burn calories and strengthen your heart.

Before I recommend some cardiovascular activities, let me briefly explain what cardiovascular fitness is. It is the ability and efficiency of your lungs, heart, and vascular system to transport oxygen to your muscles. Aerobic exercise strengthens cardiovascular fitness. *Aerobic* means with, or in the presence of, oxygen. Walking, jogging, and biking are all examples of aerobic exercises—exercises that utilize oxygen. Incorporating aerobic exercise into your life will improve your cardiovascular fitness because your body learns to utilize its oxygen supply more efficiently. When you utilize oxygen more efficiently, your heart works less to pump blood and oxygen throughout your body. This results in a stronger, more efficient heart.

Who wants to walk down the aisle and appear out of breath? And let's not forget the reception! It will be an utter embarrassment if you can't do the electric slide and macarena back to back!

For most brides, shedding a few pounds is important. During aerobic exercise, your body expends a lot of energy because you utilize and process more oxygen. This energy is measured in calories. For every liter of oxygen used during an aerobic activity (per kilogram of body weight), the body spends five calories. The more energy you spend and the longer you exercise, the more oxygen is used and the more calories you will burn. I encourage brides-to-be to exercise longer at a lower intensity to maintain current weight or lose a few pounds.

CARDIOVASCULAR ACTIVITIES

Walking (with a Purpose!)

Walking is a low-impact activity. It is inexpensive, easy, and convenient. Yet in today's fast-paced world, people don't walk anymore! We are obsessed with convenience and getting from point A to point B as quickly as possible. Slow down, get out of the car, and use walking as an effective exercise tool! Instead of hailing a cab, catching a bus, or driving to the local deli, walk there—and walk with a purpose. Elevate that heart rate! Walking can be done anywhere. Check out your neighborhood, walk to do your errands, or even be part of the mall walkers' cult!

If you choose walking as part of your cardiovascular routine, invest in a decent pair of walking shoes. Make sure your posture is good and your feet move smoothly from heel to toe. Swinging your arms will help elevate your heart rate as well. Your arms should counter your legs. If you are a beginner, start walking for about ten minutes at a brisk pace. Gradually increase your time and speed. Over time you will be able to increase your time to thirty minutes to one hour, every other day to every day.

Jogging/Running

One of the most popular aerobic activities, running is a great way to burn calories and strengthen the cardiovascular system. Running is easy and can be done anywhere. Again, I recommend investing in a good pair of running shoes. Don't think you have to go with the latest craze and buy the $150 pair of neon, air-induced, water-inflated sneakers that light up with each step! A good pair of running shoes will run you (no pun intended!) anywhere from $50 to $75. I suggest going to a store that specializes in running shoes. Here, a qualified specialist (usually a runner!) can assess your size and running gait, whether you pronate (your toes turn out) or supinate (your toes turn in), whether your arch is high or low, and, most important, whether the shoes fit!

Proper running clothes are important. In cold weather, make sure to layer your clothes, with "breathable" fabrics that absorb perspiration and moisture near the skin. Be sure to cover your head and ears, as this is where you lose most of your body heat. Also, it is important to wear gloves or mittens to keep your hands warm and protected.

In hot, humid weather, make sure you hydrate before a run. Drink a lot of water, wear light-colored, breathable clothing, and make sure to take a water bottle with you!

As with walking, start slowly, keeping the mileage low at first. If you run too quickly and too far, you might create a whole slew of problems. Pains and strains in the knees, Achilles tendons, quadriceps, and hamstrings are a result of too much running, too soon. As previously discussed, stretching before and after you run is a must! It is also important to run on alternate days in order to rest the body.

A few pointers for proper running technique:

- Focus on your posture: your abdominals should be pulled in, your shoulders relaxed.

- Keep your arms close to your body. Swinging your arms wildly will only use up energy. Your hands should be close to the middle of your body.

- Run from heel to toe with a comfortable stride length. Don't land flat-footed!

Biking

I like walking and running because they require the smallest amount of equipment. Biking is a great cardiovascular exercise, but of course it requires a bike! I'm not suggesting that every bride-to-be purchase a bike, but if you have one, use it!

There are two ways to ride a bike. One is to bike around leisurely, taking in the neighborhood sights. Yes, you'll have a lovely time, but you'll miss out on the aerobic conditioning of biking. The second way is to ride with intensity for speed, time, and distance. Here you not only get the aerobic benefits but you also tone and condition the muscles of the lower body.

Pages could be written on proper bike-riding technique. Basically, make sure the bike fits you. That means your feet should reach the pedals comfortably with a slight bend at the knee at full leg extension. If you have to reach for the pedals with your toes, you must adjust the seat.

There are many types of bikes, and you can outfit yours with numerous pieces of equipment. Again, do whatever it will take to motivate you to ride with intensity. I do insist, however, that you purchase a bike helmet. I've seen too many serious injuries that could have been prevented had the rider worn a helmet. Besides, you are preparing for your wedding day; don't take any chances!

Cross-Training

Cross-training is a great way to stay motivated. Cross-training involves including different aerobic exercises in your cardiovascular program. Doing the same aerobic activity for six months creates boredom Cross-training is also beneficial because you are "fooling" your body; it doesn't have the chance to adapt to one specific exercise. If, for example, you just run, your body gets used to the idea and, after a period of time, "plateaus." After a while, you don't burn as many calories because your muscles have become used to the activity. By mixing activities, you trick your body and therefore maximize the benefits of your cardiovascular program.

EXAMPLES OF A CROSS-TRAINING ROUTINE

WEEK I						
MON	TUE	WED	THU	FRI	SAT	SUN
Run	Power walk	Off	Bike	Power walk	Run	Off

WEEK II						
MON	TUE	WED	THU	FRI	SAT	SUN
Bike	Run	Power walk	Off	Bike	Run	Off

As you begin to incorporate cardiovascular exercises into your Buff Brides workout, keep your goal (and wedding date) in mind and focus. Just remember: make it fun, elevate your heart rate, and be consistent! That's all you will need to look and feel your best on that special day.

STRENGTH TRAINING

Strength training often gets a bad rap from women. The question I am asked most frequently is "Will I bulk up if I lift weights?" Time and again, I tell my clients that it is nearly impossible for women to "bulk up" when strength training. Unless you decide to set up house in the nearest gym and lift heavy weights twenty-four hours a day, you will not get bulky. Generally, women do not produce enough testosterone to "beef up."

Strength training is an important part of weight management and weight loss. Strength training develops muscular strength and endurance, helps prevent osteoporosis, reduces body fat, and improves your everyday life. With consistent weight training, your metabolic rate will increase, thereby increasing the number of calories you burn while at rest. Strength training develops the shape of your muscles and defines them. This does not mean bulk, ladies! It simply means being well toned. If looking good in your wedding dress is important to you, a consistent strength training program is imperative.

In Part II, I take you through an easy, manageable approach to strength training. I have found these exercises effective for many of the different cuts of wedding dresses on the market.

Before you strength train, always warm up. Do at least five minutes of an aerobic activity and then stretch before lifting weights.

Use weights that are not too heavy so that you can do 8 to 12 repetitions with good form. Your last repetition should be challenging. Start with one set of each exercise and, in general, work up to three sets. Proper form is mandatory! After a couple of sessions, if you feel good and experience minimal soreness, increase the weight. Continue this approach until you feel challenged toward the end of the set. In general, work larger muscle groups first. Abdominal strengthening should always be done last in your workout. Tired-out abdominals will prevent you from keeping good form during your workout.

Breathing is also important while strength training. The rule of thumb is to exhale on the lift and inhale as you lower the weight. Concentrate on the muscle you're working on. Focusing on a specific muscle will make your workouts more intense, challenging, and effective.

NUTRITION

E ating right while planning your wedding can be difficult. This stressful time in your life can lead to unbalanced eating habits. Of course, the resources available on this subject are endless. It seems as if there is a new diet/nutrition fad every day, and they often conflict with one another. And let's not forget about the nutrition stores stocked with powders, energy bars, pills, and supplements. Who can keep up with it all?

I will outline some nutrition basics that will enhance your workouts. It is imperative that the bride-to-be balance a healthy nutrition plan with her workouts. Don't try to starve yourself in order to get into your gown. Not eating properly will only *lower* your metabolism. Basically, your body will slow down its metabolism because it senses that it is being starved. Starving yourself will leave you feeling lethargic and unmotivated.

Everyone's body is different. Some people naturally have a higher metabolism than others. While incorporating the Buff Brides workout into your lifestyle, try to track what you eat and see how it affects your workouts. You may need to experiment a little to determine what works best for you.

A question many of my clients ask is "How many calories should I eat?" That depends on factors such as your body type, weight, height, and genetic makeup. If your goal is to lose weight, record everything you eat for a few days and add up the calories. The number of calories you consume each day may surprise you.

The rule of thumb is that you must reduce your caloric intake by about 3,500 calories to lose one pound of weight. Roughly, if you cut 500 calories per day from your diet or burn an extra 500 calories per day through exercise, you should lose about a pound per week. Again I stress that an exercise program complemented by a healthy eating plan will yield quicker and healthier weight loss. Losing more than one pound a week is not only unhealthy, it is usually ineffective, as most people gain this weight back.

Balancing Carbohydrates, Protein, and Fat

This is another piece of the nutrition puzzle that is often debated. I believe that a healthy balance of all three works best. Carbohydrates and fats are crucial for giving your body energy, and proteins are important for building and repairing muscles. Again, everyone's body is different, but you should get roughly 50 to 60 percent of your calories from carbohydrates (one gram of carbohydrates contains 4 calories), 15 to 20 percent of your calories from proteins (one gram of protein contains 4 calories), and 20 to 30 percent of your calories from fat (one gram of fat contains 9 calories). To see optimum results from your Buff Brides workout, consuming a balanced diet and enough calories without starving yourself is crucial!

Don't Forget the Water!

A bride-to-be can never get enough water. When exercising, you need plenty of water to cool your body, carry nutrients to your cells, and carry waste to your kidneys. Most people drink water only when they are thirsty. Don't wait to feel thirsty to drink water, as you may already be on your way to dehydration. Eight to ten glasses of water a day is recommended, more if you are exercising.

Another common question is "Should I eat before I work out?" Yes! Food is the fuel that runs your body. That's not to say you should eat a huge meal before working out, but if you haven't eaten for hours before a workout, you'll run out of energy! If you're working out during the wee hours of the morning, you should at least eat something high in carbohydrates. Eating after a workout is important too, as you need to replenish the nutrients lost while working out. Drinking plenty of water and other fluids after a workout is also important.

BODY TYPES/DRESSES

Just like wedding dresses, brides come in many different sizes. You might think the opposite, what with all the bridal magazines emphasizing the statuesque 5-foot, 11-inch bride! The shocking truth is that there is more out there than size eights. The bad news is that your body build is pretty much determined when you are born. The good news is that you can change the amount of fat versus the amount of muscle you have in your body. But in order to do that you must incorporate exercise and good eating habits into your life.

The three basic body types are ectomorph, endomorph, and mesomorph. Ectomorphs are usually long and thin. Their bone structure is usually delicate. Ectomorphs are lightly muscled and sometimes have trouble gaining weight.

Mesomorphs are bigger-boned. They usually gain muscle easily. Their shoulders are often wider than their hips. Mesomorphs are often referred to as "medium build." If people with this body type eat improperly, they tend to gain weight.

Endomorphs are often referred to as "pear-shaped," as their hips are often wider than their shoulders. This body type tends to hold fat more, thus making it harder for them to lose weight.

I have worked with all three of these common body types. When choosing a gown, work with your body type. Feel good when making this important decision!

The Slim Bride (Ectomorph)

The slim bride looks best in A-lines and sheath gowns. Slim brides should stay away from bouffant skirts, as they may get lost! Dresses that emphasize detailing at the neckline help draw the eyes up to the face. Taller headpieces can also add height. Slim brides also look fabulous in strapless and off-the-shoulder styles.

The Full-Figured Bride (Mesomorph)

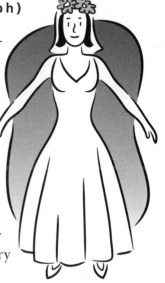

A full-figured bride should try to avoid bulky fabrics such as velvets and satins. Instead, she should consider lighter, softer fabrics such as silks and chiffons. She should try to de-emphasize the neckline by choosing a dress with a V neck or scoop neck. Fitted sleeves are better than puffed or full sleeves. Empire waists and A-lines work well for the full-figured bride, as do ball gowns with a basque waist. Full-figured brides should stay away from mermaid and form-fitting sheath silhouettes. Headpieces and jewelry draw attention to the face.

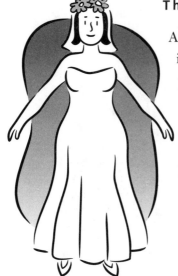

The Pear-Shaped Bride (Endomorph)

A strapless ball gown works best for this type of bride, as it places the focus on the upper part of the body. A pear-shaped bride should avoid a V neck and opt for an off-the-shoulder neckline, which makes the upper half of the body look more proportional to the lower half.

PART II

The Exercises

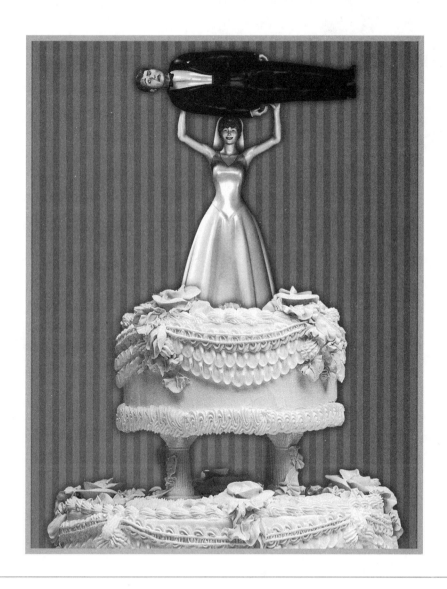

LEGS AND BUTT

Although most styles of wedding dresses emphasize the upper body, it is still crucial to tone and strengthen the legs and butt. There are hundreds of exercises that work the lower body; however, I feel the following ones are some of the best. Many of these exercises utilize an exercise ball. These exercises are a must for brides who get cold feet on their wedding day and need to do a quick sprint before the ceremony begins!

"Quality Quads" (Quadriceps Muscles)

The quadriceps are some of the largest muscles in your body. They comprise the muscles on the front of your thigh. The quads are a group of four different muscles: the rectus femoris, vastus lateralis, vastus medialis, and vastus intermedialis. The rectus femoris runs along the front of your thigh, crossing both your hip and knee joints. It flexes your hip and extends your knee. Strong quads are especially useful during the reception when you are forced to do the hustle with Uncle Larry!

WALL SITS WITH EXERCISE BALL

For this exercise, you need a sturdy wall and an exercise ball. Standing up, place the exercise ball behind your lower back, between you and the wall. Make sure your feet are shoulder width apart, your heels pressed firmly into the floor.

Slowly bend your knees into a squatting position, letting the ball roll toward the middle of your back. Make sure your back is straight, your abdominals are tight, and you are looking straight ahead. It may help to look into a mirror in order to ensure perfect form. While squatting, make sure your knees stay over your toes and keep your hands at your sides. Squat until you are in a

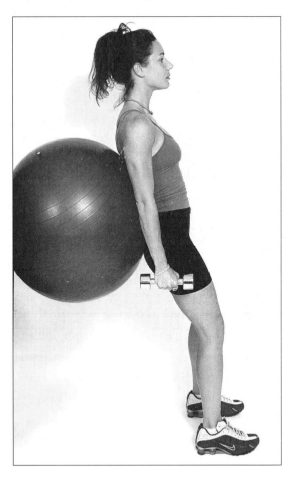

sitting position, then slowly come back up, pushing your heels into the floor, and return to the original position. Do not lock your knees when standing up. Inhale on the way down and exhale on the way up. For added resistance, hold a 3- to 5-pound dumbbell in each hand, keeping them steady at your sides.

BEGINNER

No weights • 8–12 repetitions • 1–2 sets

INTERMEDIATE/ADVANCED

3–5-lb. dumbbells • 12–15 repetitions • 3 sets

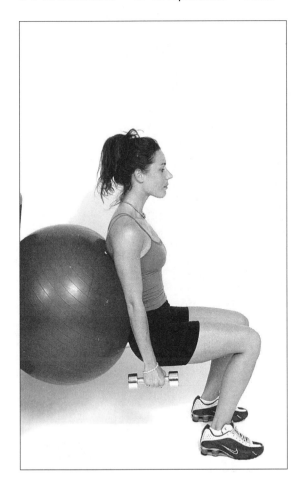

DUMBBELL LUNGES

Stand with a dumbbell in each hand, your arms at your sides. Keeping your back straight and your feet shoulder width apart, step forward with your left foot, slightly more than you would when taking a normal step. Your upper body should remain upright and your arms should remain steady at your sides, dumbbells staying toward the center of your body.

Your left leg should be bent at a 90-degree angle; your knee should be over your toes. Your right leg should be slightly bent

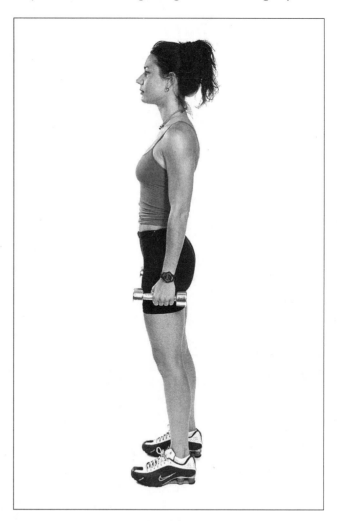

as you lunge forward, and your heel will rise slightly. Return to the starting position and repeat with your right foot.

No weights • 8–12 repetitions • 1–2 sets

INTERMEDIATE/ADVANCED

3–5-lb. dumbbells • 12–15 repetitions • 2–3 sets

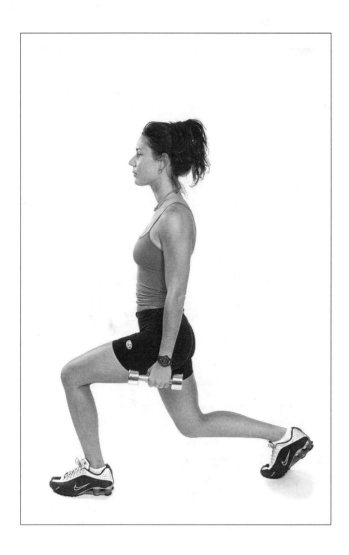

DUMBBELL STEP-UPS

Stand upright with a dumbbell in each hand, palms facing in. Your chest should be out, your abdominals in, your shoulders back. Stand in front of a step or box 12 to 15 inches high and about a foot away.

Place your right foot on the center of the step. Shifting your weight to that foot, step up onto the top of the step, bringing both feet together to the center of the step. Keep the dumbbells steady at your sides and your shoulders relaxed.

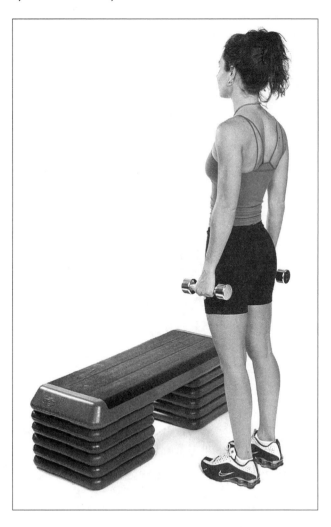

Step backward, left foot first, then follow with your right foot. Repeat the exercise, leading with your left foot.

BEGINNER

3–5-lb. dumbbells • 8–12 repetitions • 1–2 sets

INTERMEDIATE/ADVANCED

5–10-lb. dumbbells • 12–15 repetitions • 2–3 sets

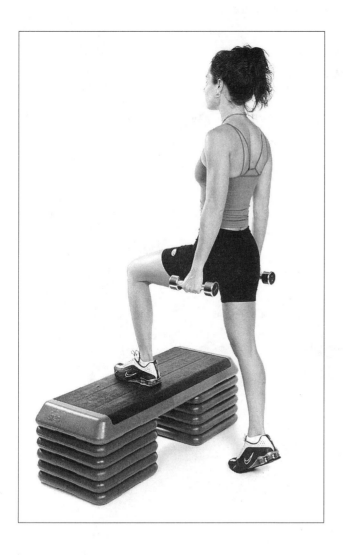

Abductor Muscles

The abductor muscles are in the outer part of the thigh and butt. Most women feel that this is one of their bigger "problem areas." Women naturally tend to store fat on their hips, and this portion of the body is often lovingly referred to as "saddlebags." Toning and defining this area are always priorities for the bride-to-be. After all, the only luggage you'll want to carry is the suitcase you're taking on your honeymoon!

LYING BENT-LEG SIDE RAISES

When performing this exercise, it is important to use an inverted (in-rotated) foot position on the leg you're training. This allows the leg to rotate in, which then focuses the work on the outside of the leg.

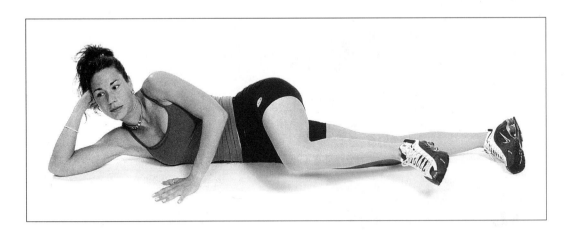

Lie on your side with your bottom leg bent, top leg straight out, foot rotated in. Support your head on your outstretched arm and stabilize your body by placing your other hand on the floor in front of your chest.

On the count of four, lift your top leg as high as you can without twisting your torso or arching your back. Keeping your leg controlled, return to the starting position to the count of four. After one set, repeat with the other leg.

BEGINNER

No weights • 8–12 repetitions • 1–2 sets

INTERMEDIATE/ADVANCED

3–5-lb. ankle weights • 12–15 repetitions • 2–3 sets

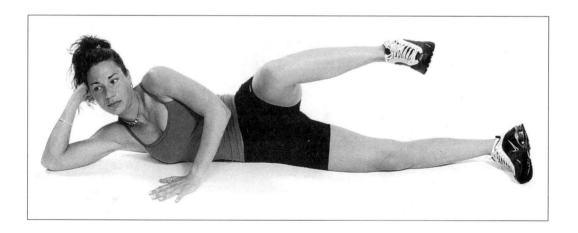

Adductor Muscles

The adductor muscles are in the inner part of the thigh. These muscles are opposite the abductor muscles.

LYING ADDUCTIONS

An everted, or out-rotated, position is best when performing this exercise. This allows the leg to rotate out, which then focuses the movement on the inside of the leg.

Lie on your back with your left leg extended. Your right leg is bent, foot flat on the floor. Your left leg should be

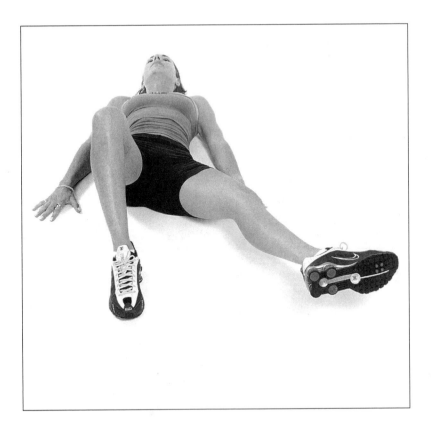

stretched away from your right leg and slightly raised off the floor.

On the count of four, leading with the heel, pull your left foot in until it is even with your right foot. Maintaining control, return to the starting position to the count of four. After one set, repeat with the right leg.

BEGINNER

No weights • 8–12 repetitions • 1–2 sets

INTERMEDIATE/ADVANCED

3–5-lb. ankle weights • 12–15 repetitions • 2–3 sets

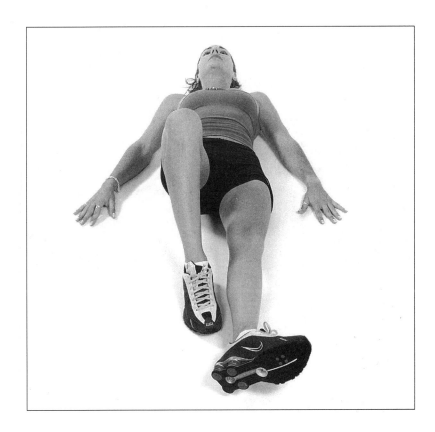

Hamstring Muscles

The hamstring muscles are located behind your thighs. Flexible, well-conditioned hamstrings form a defined curve down the back of your upper leg.

LEG CURLS WITH EXERCISE BALL

Lie on your back with an exercise ball under your heels and the lower portion of your legs. Your arms should be at your sides, palms toward the ground.

Lift your hips/pelvis up as high as you can. On the count of four, roll the ball toward your butt, using your lower legs and heels. At first you may find it hard to stabilize yourself. This will

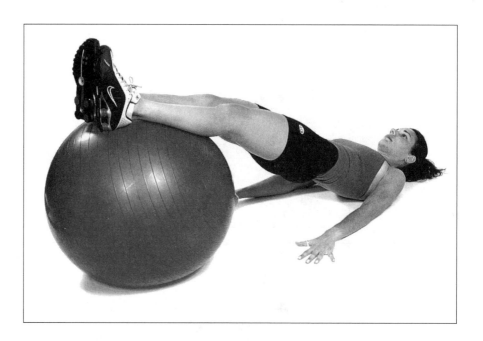

improve once your core/abdominal strength improves. Once the ball is almost touching your butt, return to the starting position to the count of four. Don't drop your hips throughout the set.

Exhale as you roll the ball toward you; *inhale* as you return to the starting position.

BEGINNER

8–12 repetitions • 1 set

INTERMEDIATE/ADVANCED

10–12 repetitions • 2–3 sets

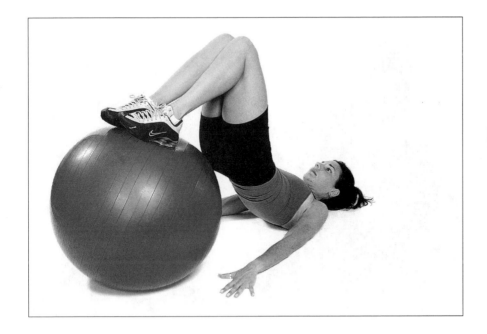

THE TONED, TRIMMED BUTT!

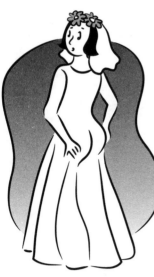

It doesn't matter what style of dress you choose, the butt is certainly one of the focal areas for any bride-to-be. The butt muscles are some of the largest muscles in your body, so toning this part of your body is crucial. Your butt muscles come in three sizes: the gluteus maximus, gluteus medius, and gluteus minimus. The maximus, as the name implies, is the largest group and more noticeable than the medius and minimus. The following exercises are devised to tone your glutei maximi and by no means make them as big as your wedding cake!

BUTT LIFTS WITH EXERCISE BALL

Lie on your back on the floor with your heels on an exercise ball, feet slightly apart. Your toes should be pointing toward the ceiling. Your arms should be at your sides, palms facedown.

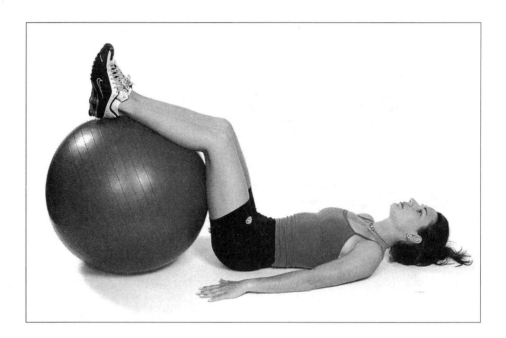

Exhale as you lift your pelvis toward the ceiling; *inhale* as you return to the starting position.

Counting to four, lift your pelvis toward the ceiling. Squeeze your butt muscles together as you lift until your back is straight. Don't arch your back or push yourself up with your hands. Keeping your butt muscles tight, return to the starting position to the count of four. As you return to the starting position, don't rest your butt on the floor.

BEGINNER

8–12 repetitions • 2 sets

INTERMEDIATE/ADVANCED

12–15 repetitions • 2–3 sets

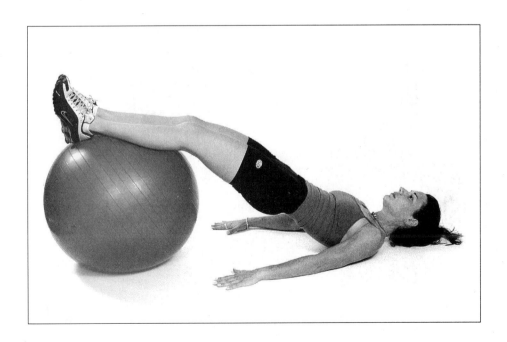

STANDING KICKBACKS

Standing, face a wall and extend your arms, placing your hands on the wall for support. Your hips should be squarely facing the wall, your feet shoulder width apart. Lean forward slightly so your body is in a straight line.

Shift your weight to your right leg and, to the count of four, move your left leg back as far as you can. Maintain good position by not arching your back. As you move the leg back, tighten your butt muscles so you feel the contraction. Return to

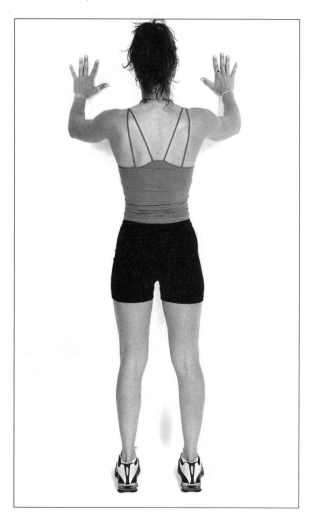

the starting position to the count of four, maintaining the contraction. After one set, switch legs.

3–5-lb. ankle weights • 8–12 repetitions • 2–3 sets

5–10-lb. ankle weights • 12–15 repetitions • 3 sets

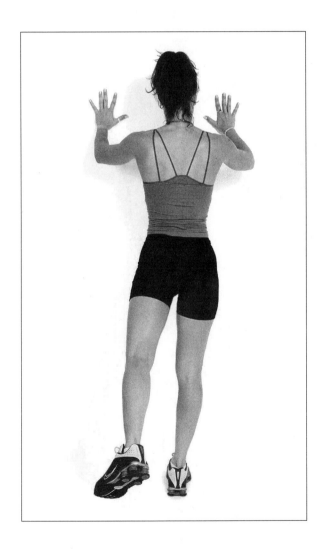

BENT-LEG KICKBACKS

Get down on all fours, your back flat, your head aligned with your spine. Your hands should be shoulder width apart. Look at the floor.

Keeping your foot flexed throughout the movement, raise your right leg back and up, at a 90-degree angle, pointing the sole of your foot toward the ceiling. As you lift up, squeeze your butt muscles together, but don't arch your back. Bring the leg

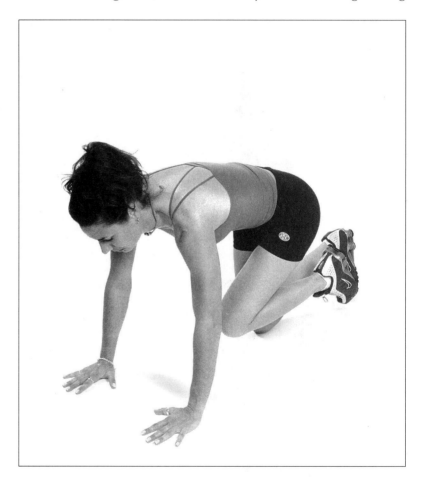

forward until the knee is almost touching the chest and repeat.
After one set, switch legs.

BEGINNER

3-lb. ankle weights • 8–12 repetitions • 2–3 sets

INTERMEDIATE/ADVANCED

5–8-lb. ankle weights • 12–15 repetitions • 2–3 sets

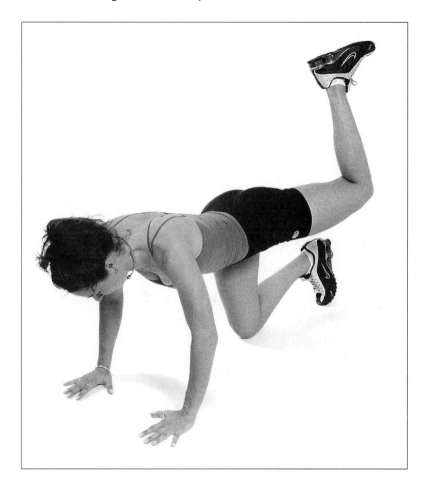

Many of today's wedding dresses emphasize the back. Some are cut low, while others reveal the back through lace. Most women neglect to develop the muscles in the back because they can't see them. A toned back will make you appear leaner, allow you to stand taller, and make you look beautiful as you take your vows at the altar!

BACK EXTENSIONS ON EXERCISE BALL

Kneel behind an exercise ball and place your hands behind your back. Lean forward and lengthen your body and straighten your legs so that your torso/midsection is resting

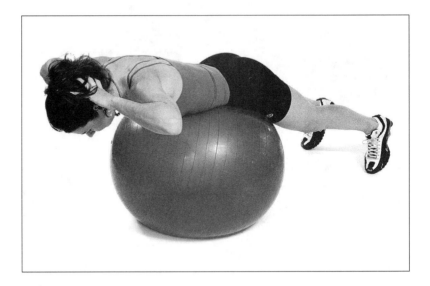

firmly against the ball. Your toes should remain on the ground to maintain balance. Place your hands behind your head, fingers interlocked.

To the count of four, lift your chest upward just a few inches. Keep your head steady and your elbows out. Slowly lower your chest to the starting position, to the count of four.

BEGINNER

8–12 repetitions • 1 set

INTERMEDIATE/ADVANCED

12–15 repetitions • 2–3 sets

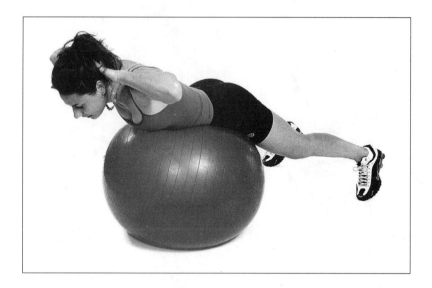

ONE-ARM DUMBBELL ROWS

Place your right knee on the center of a bench or a sturdy coffee table. Your right hand should be braced on the bench or table. Your weight should be resting on your right knee and hand. Pick up a dumbbell in your left hand, palm facing toward you. Your left foot should be firmly on the ground. Your back should be as straight as possible.

Lift the dumbbell up and in to the count of four. Lead with the elbow and raise the weight as high as you can toward your

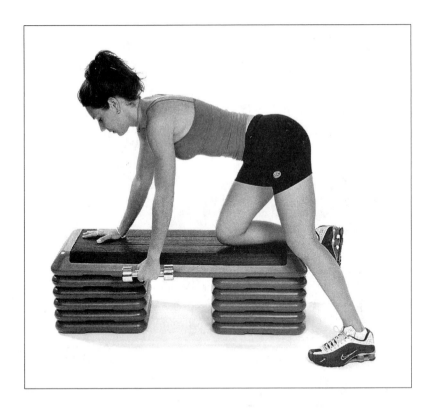

chest muscles. Lower your arm to the starting position to the count of four. After one set, reverse position and repeat on the other side.

BEGINNER

3–5-lb. dumbbells • 12–15 repetitions • 1 set

INTERMEDIATE/ADVANCED

5–10-lb. dumbbells • 12–15 repetitions • 2–3 sets

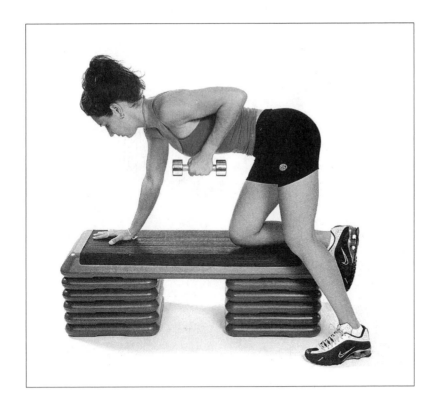

SUPERBRIDES

Lie facedown on an exercise mat or carpet. Extend your legs, toes pointed. Extend your arms over your head. Look forward, keeping your head steady, your chin off the ground.

Slowly raise your left arm and right leg at the same time until they are a few inches off the ground. Slowly lower to starting position. Repeat with your right arm and left leg.

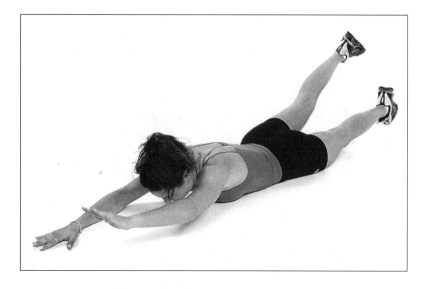

12–15 repetitions • 1 set

12–15 repetitions • 2–3 sets

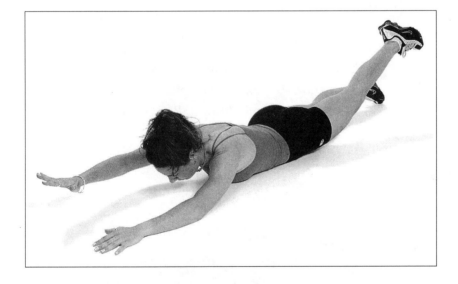

"Perky Pecs" (Pectoral Muscles)

Many of the wedding gowns today have open necklines that make the chest more visible. Scoop-necked, Empire, sheath, and historical are just some of the basic bridal silhouettes that emphasize the chest. A firm, well-toned bust will add lift as well as improve your posture when you are walking down the aisle. Gown makers will encourage you to show off your chest. Here are a few sure-fire exercises to make sure Grandma's diamond necklace will look its best.

CHEST PRESS

For this exercise, you will need an exercise ball or sturdy bench. If you are using a ball, lie back on the ball so your head and neck are stabilized by it. Push your hips up so that

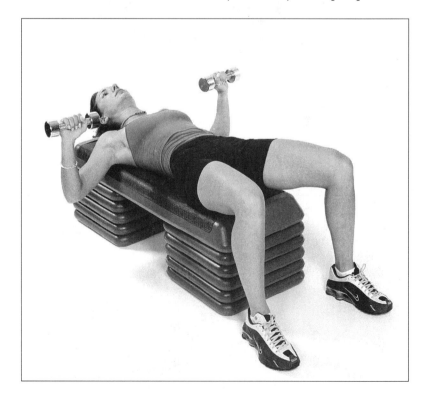

your abdominal and butt muscles are tight. If you are using a bench, put it in the flat position and lie down pressing your lower back into it. Keep your abdominals and butt muscles tight. Pick up a dumbbell in each hand and hold them above you, with your palms facing out. Keep the dumbbells shoulder width apart. Don't allow your hips to drop, as you are also strengthening the core muscles with this exercise. To the count of four, slowly lower the dumbbells until they are even with your chest. Raise them to the starting position to the count of four. Exhale on the exertion (when you push up) and inhale when lowering the dumbbells.

BEGINNER

5–10-lb. dumbbells • 12–15 repetitions • 1 set

INTERMEDIATE/ADVANCED

10–15-lb. dumbbells • 12–15 repetitions • 2–3 sets

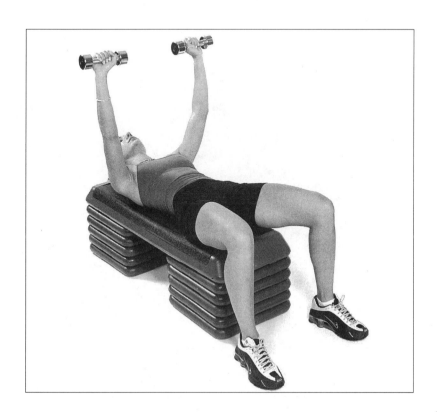

PUSH-UPS ON EXERCISE BALL

Get into a push-up position with an exercise ball under your knees. Keep your back straight, hands shoulder width apart, thumbs pointing toward each other. Keep your elbows straight but not locked. Keep your abdominal muscles contracted so that your midsection is stabilized throughout the exercise. To the count of four, bend your elbows and lower your chest to the floor. Push up to the starting position to the count of four. Don't place your hands too wide or too narrow, and don't lead with your hips.

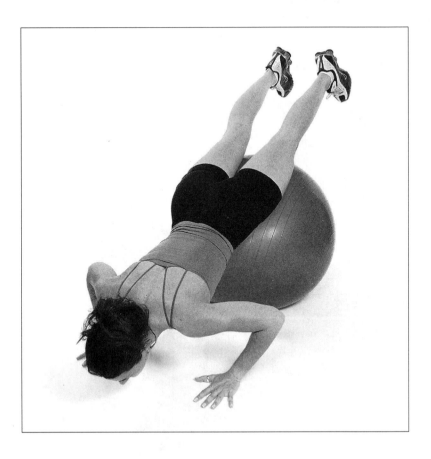

Inhale as you lower your chest to the floor; *exhale* as you return to the starting position.

BEGINNER

8–10 repetitions • 1 set

INTERMEDIATE/ADVANCED

10–12 repetitions • 2–3 sets

FITNESS TIP

*I*ncrease the intensity of the exercise by placing the ball closer to your feet. Placing the ball more toward the midline of your body will make the exercise easier.

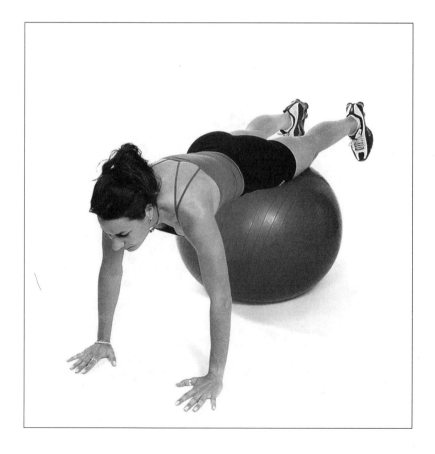

Shoulders

Good posture is imperative when walking down the aisle. Pulling back your shoulders and walking tall will allow you to really show off your wedding dress. Most dresses expose the shoulders, and one of the most common requests I get from brides-to-be is for "cut and toned" shoulders. The deltoids define most of the shoulder area. To achieve optimum height on your bouquet toss, strong delts are a must!

SEATED OVERHEAD PRESS

Sit on the edge of a sturdy chair, feet flat on the floor. You may also sit on an exercise ball, but be sure to keep your abs tight and your back straight. Hold two dumbbells just in front of

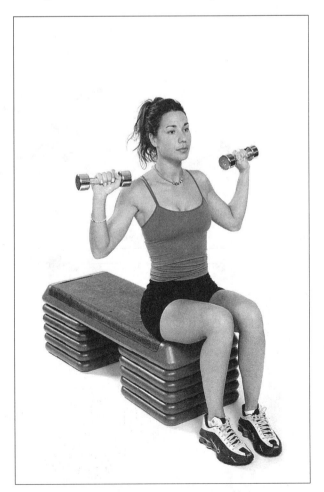

your shoulders, palms facing out. Look straight ahead. If you have a mirror, use it so you can keep an eye on your form.

To the count of four, extend your arms and lift the dumbbells above your head. The dumbbells should gently touch each other at the extension. Pause and lower the dumbbells to your shoulders, again to the count of four. Envision making a triangle from start to finish. Don't lock your elbows or arch your back. The movement should be smooth.

BEGINNER

3–5-lb. dumbbells • 8–12 repetitions • 1 set

INTERMEDIATE/ADVANCED

5–10-lb. dumbbells • 12–15 repetitions • 2–3 sets

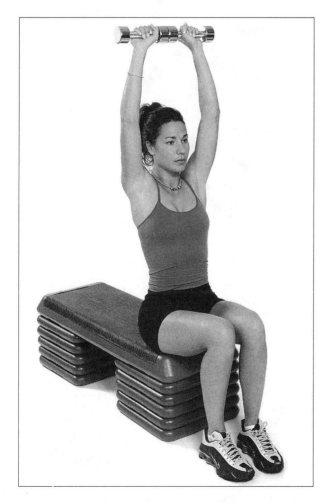

LATERAL RAISES

Standing, hold two dumbbells at your sides, your palms facing your body. Keep your lower back straight and lean forward slightly. Keep your abdominals tight, feet shoulder width apart.

Keep your elbows bent at a 90° angle. To the count of four, raise both dumbbells out to the sides, and up to shoulder height. Lower the dumbbells to the starting position to the

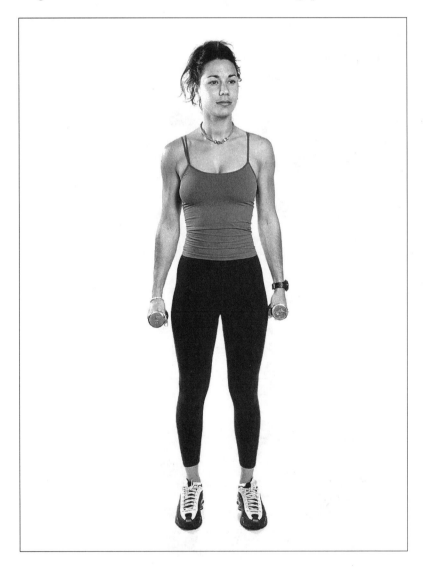

count of four. Don't raise the dumbbells above shoulder height, and don't lock your knees.

BEGINNER

3–5-lb. dumbbells • 8–12 repetitions • 1 set

INTERMEDIATE/ADVANCED

5–10-lb. dumbbells • 12–15 repetitions • 2–3 sets

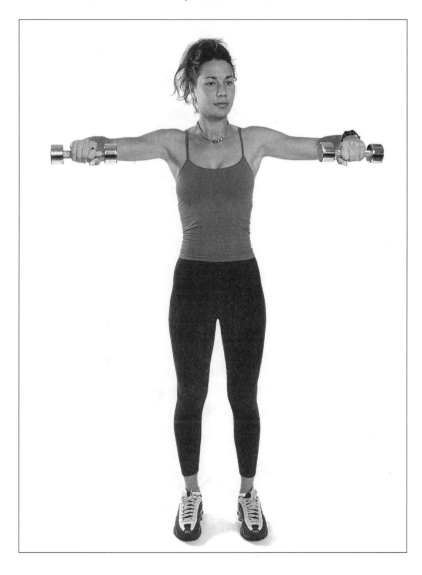

ALTERNATING FRONT RAISES

Standing, with your feet shoulder width apart, hold two dumbbells in front of you, your palms facing your body. Keep your shoulders back, your lower back straight, and your body slightly leaning forward. Keep your abdominal muscles tight. To the count of four, raise one dumbbell until it is at shoulder height. Pause, then lower the dumbbell to the starting position to the count of four. Repeat, using the other arm. Don't

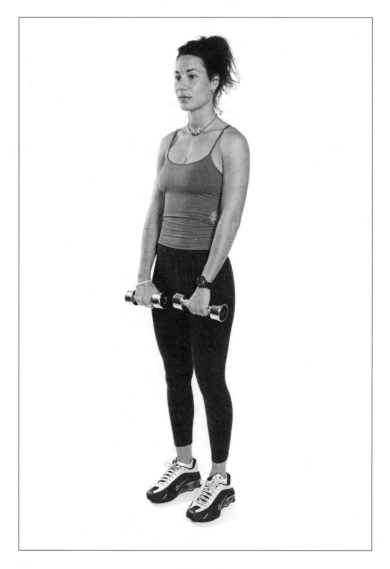

arch your back, and don't raise the dumbbell above shoulder height.

3–5-lb. dumbbells • 8–12 repetitions • 1 set

5–10-lb. dumbbells • 12–15 repetitions • 2–3 sets

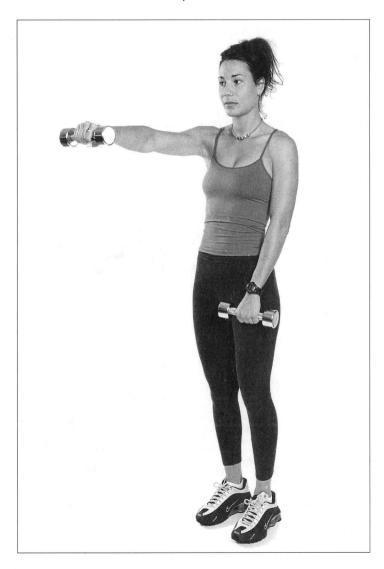

"Tricky Tris" (Triceps)

"When feeding my husband the wedding cake, I *do not* want the guests staring at my flabby arm!" This is a common statement from the panicked brides-to-be I train. We've all seen wedding videos of the "waving wattle"! Brides, relax. By doing the following exercises, you will make the muscle that runs along the back of your upper arm a work of art, not a photo nightmare!

TRICEPS KICKBACKS

Using a sturdy chair, place your right knee on the chair seat for support. (The edge of a coffee table will also do.) Pick up a dumbbell in your left hand, palm facing your body. Your right

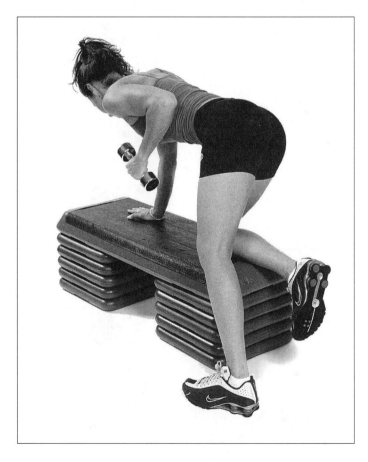

hand is reaching forward on the chair seat for support. Your left foot is flat on the ground.

Keeping your left arm close to your rib cage, extend the dumbbell back and away from your body to the count of four, until your arm is straight and parallel to the floor and your palm is facing your torso. Tighten your triceps at the end of the motion. Lower your arm to the starting position to the count of four. Don't arch your back, and keep your head bent forward.

BEGINNER

3–5-lb. dumbbells • 8–12 repetitions • 1 set

INTERMEDIATE/ADVANCED

5–8-lb. dumbbells • 10–12 repetitions • 2–3 sets

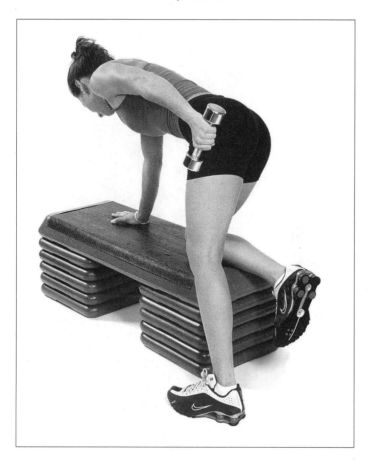

TRICEPS DIPS

Sit on a chair with your hands gripping the edge of the seat (again, a sturdy coffee table can also be used). Your legs should be bent and your feet flat on the floor. With your legs together, move forward until your hips and butt are off the seat.

On the count of four, slowly lower your hips toward the floor until your arms are bent at a 90-degree angle. Keep your butt close to the chair. Return to the starting position, where

FITNESS TIP

*A*t first you may not be able to achieve a 90-degree angle. In that case, simply lower yourself as far as your muscles will allow.

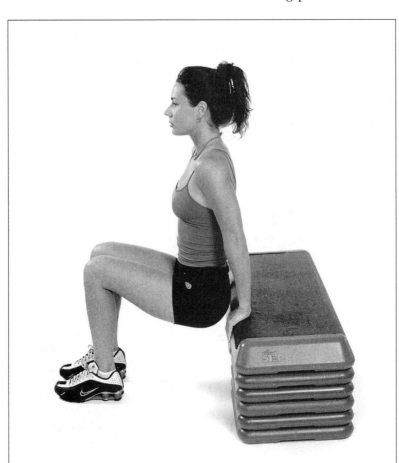

your arms are at full extension, to the count of four. Don't lock your arms.

BEGINNER

8–10 repetitions • 1 set

INTERMEDIATE/ADVANCED

10–12 repetitions • 2–3 sets

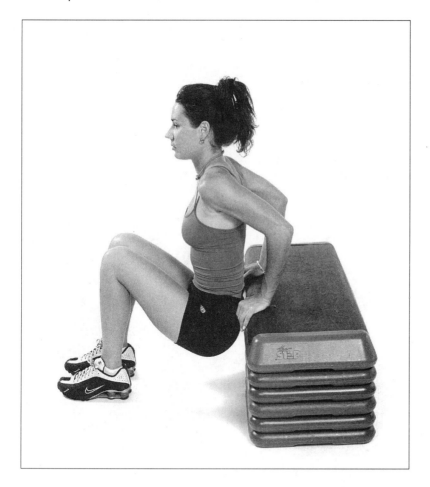

TRICEPS EXTENSIONS ON EXERCISE BALL

Lie on an exercise ball, placing it behind your head so your head and neck are stabilized. Your knees should be bent and your feet flat on the ground. Push your hips up, squeezing your glutei maximi and keeping your abdominal muscles tight.

With a dumbbell in each hand, extend your arms up, palms facing in. To the count of four, lower the dumbbells to your ears, bending at the elbows, not at the shoulders. Return to the

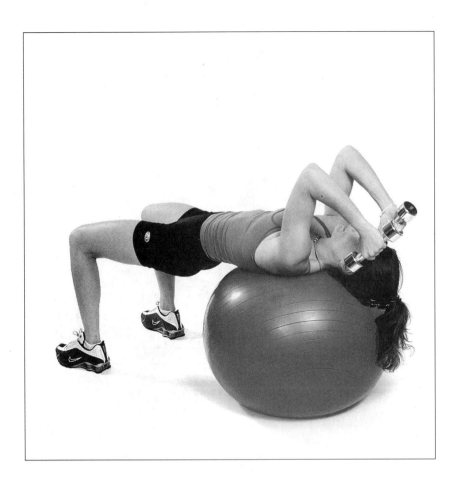

starting position to the count of four. Keep your hips pushed up during the entire exercise.

BEGINNER

3–5-lb. dumbbells • 8–12 repetitions • 1–2 sets

INTERMEDIATE/ADVANCED

5–8-lb. dumbbells • 12–15 repetitions • 2–3 sets

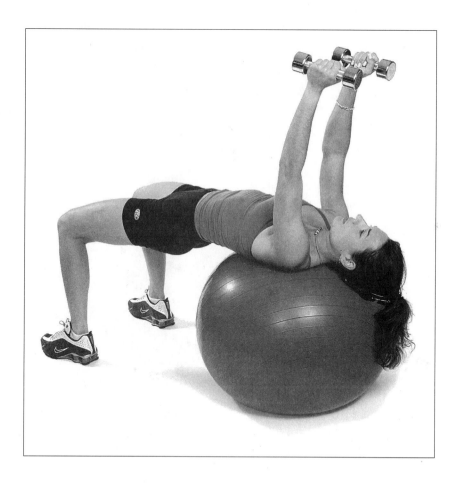

"Better Bis" (Biceps)

Having well-toned biceps does not mean you'll look like Arnold Schwarzenegger in a wedding dress. Well-toned, strong biceps are a must in all types of gown styles. The biceps, which are located opposite the triceps, will come in handy when you have to carry your husband across the threshold on your wedding night!

ALTERNATING DUMBBELL CURLS

Standing, hold a dumbbell in each hand with your arms down, your palms facing your body, and your feet shoulder width apart. Your elbows should be close to your sides.

To the count of four, curl the right-hand dumbbell up

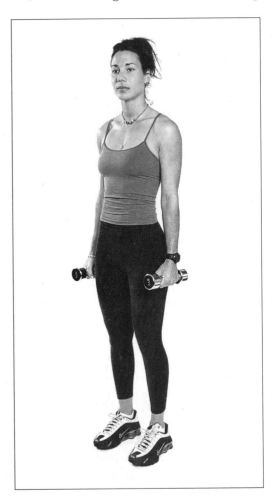

toward your right biceps, slowly turning your wrist so your palm is facing your shoulder as you finish the curl. Keep your back upright and your butt muscles tight throughout the movement. Lower to the starting position, turning your wrist back so your palm is facing your body at the bottom of the curl, to the count of four. Repeat with your left arm. Don't sway your shoulder at the beginning of the movement to gain momentum.

BEGINNER

3–5-lb. dumbbells • 8–12 repetitions • 1–2 sets

INTERMEDIATE/ADVANCED

5–10-lb. dumbbells • 12–15 repetitions • 2–3 sets

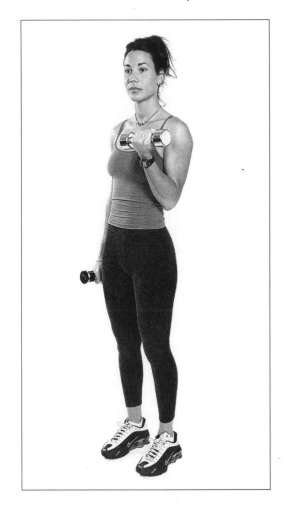

ALTERNATING HAMMER CURLS

Sitting on the edge of a chair or on an exercise ball, hold a dumbbell in each hand, arms extended down, palms facing your body, your feet flat on the floor.

To the count of four, curl the right-hand dumbbell toward your right biceps. Keep your back straight and your abdominal and butt muscles tight throughout the movement. Keep your wrist locked and your palm facing your body as you complete the lift. Lower the dumbbell to the starting position to the

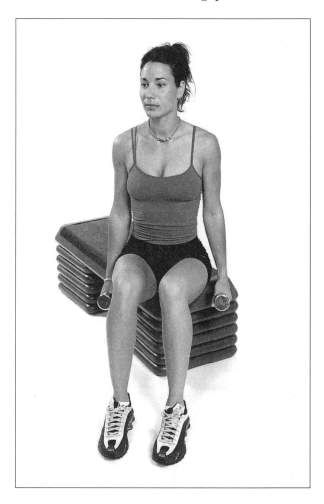

count of four, keeping the same form. Repeat with your left arm. Don't arch your back, and don't sway your shoulder at the beginning of the movement in order to gain momentum.

BEGINNER

3–5-lb. dumbbells • 8–12 repetitions • 1–2 sets

INTERMEDIATE/ADVANCED

5–10-lb. dumbbells • 12–15 repetitions • 2–3 sets

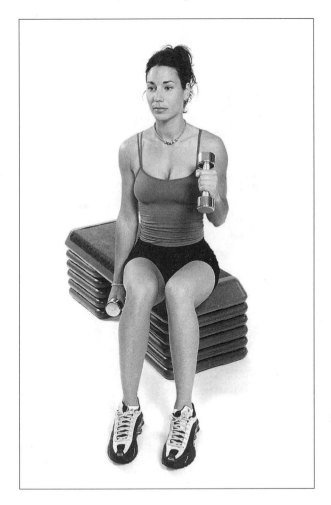

CONCENTRATION BICEPS CURLS

Sit on the edge of a chair, holding a dumbbell in your right hand. Your feet should be more than shoulder width apart so you can hold the dumbbell between your knees. Bend forward and let the dumbbell hang so your elbow is resting against your upper thigh. Your palm should be facing your left knee and your left hand resting on your left knee.

To a count of four, curl up the dumbbell until it is close to your shoulder. Pause, then lower it to the count of four. Your right elbow should remain in contact with your right knee. Do

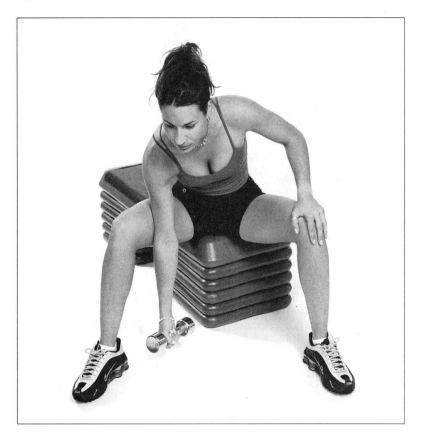

the suggested number of repetitions, then repeat with your left hand. Don't arch your back, and keep your elbow in contact with your upper thigh throughout the exercise.

BEGINNER

3–5-lb. dumbbells • 8–12 repetitions • 1 set

INTERMEDIATE/ADVANCED

5–10-lb. dumbbells • 10–12 repetitions • 2–3 sets

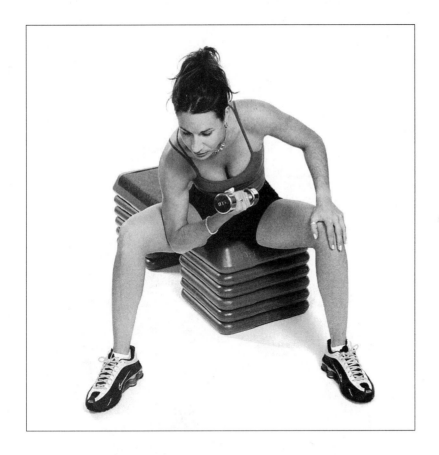

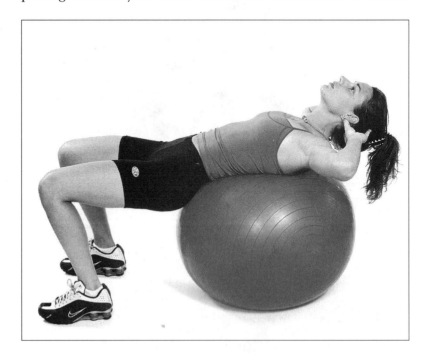

The abdominal muscles are about the only muscle group that you can work out every day. I have found that brides-to-be are very concerned about their abs because many dress styles are snug in this area. Your abdominal muscles are actually made up of several muscle groups, all located in the midsection from below your chest to past your waistline. Brides are especially concerned with their obliques, the stomach muscles that make up the waistline. There are hundreds of exercises to strengthen and tone the abdominals; I will highlight the most effective ones.

CRUNCHES ON EXERCISE BALL

Place an exercise ball on the ground and lie down on the ball, placing it under your lower back. Your feet should be flat on the floor, your hands behind your head, your thumbs under your earlobes. Keep your elbows spread wide and parallel to the floor. Focus on a point on the ceiling in order to keep your head balanced.

To the count of four, slowly curl your upper torso up and in until your shoulder blades are off the ball. Only your shoulders should lift, not your back. Feel the contraction in your abdominals and slowly return to the starting position to the count of four. Don't let your head drop back as you return.

Exhale as you curl up; *inhale* as you return to the starting position.

BEGINNER

12–15 repetitions • 3–4 sets

INTERMEDIATE/ADVANCED

15–20 repetitions • 4–5 sets

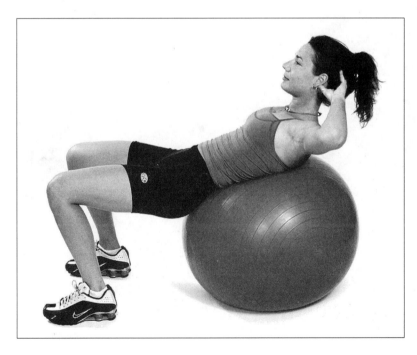

RAISED-LEG CRUNCHES ON EXERCISE BALL

Lie on your back with your legs bent over the top of the exercise ball. The ball should be behind your knees. Place your hands behind your head, thumbs under your earlobes, keeping your elbows wide.

To the count of four, lift your torso up and in toward your knees. Your shoulder blades should come off the ground. Feel the contraction in your abdominal muscles, pause, then come back down to the count of four. Don't let your abs relax as you return; repeat.

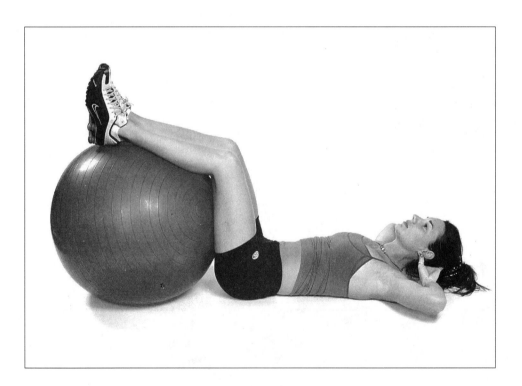

Exhale as you lift your torso toward your knees; *inhale* as you come down to the starting position.

BEGINNER

12–15 repetitions • 3–4 sets

INTERMEDIATE/ADVANCED

15–20 repetitions • 3–5 sets

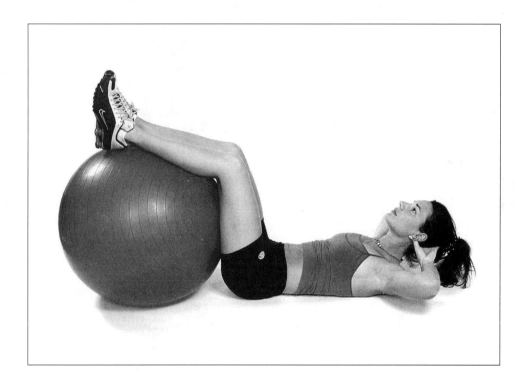

DUMBBELL SIDE BENDS

Standing, hold a dumbbell in your left hand, palm facing in. Place the palm of your right hand behind your head to stabilize it. Feet should be shoulder width apart. Don't lock your knees.

To the count of four, bend to one side, letting the dumbbell slide down the outside of your thigh. Keep your body facing forward, and don't drop your head. Go as low as you can, so that you feel the obliques (waistline muscles) working. Keep your abdominal muscles tight and contracted through-

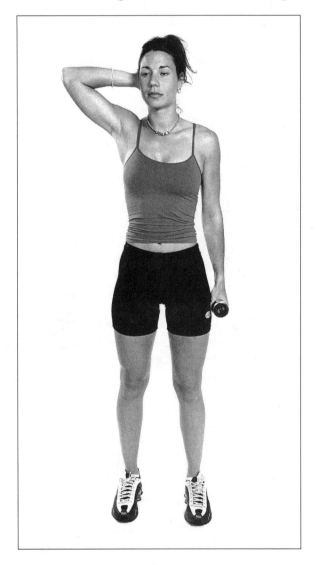

out the set. Return to the starting position to a count of four.
After one set, switch sides.

3–5-lb. dumbbells • 8–12 repetitions • 2–3 sets

5–10-lb. dumbbells • 12–15 repetitions • 3 sets

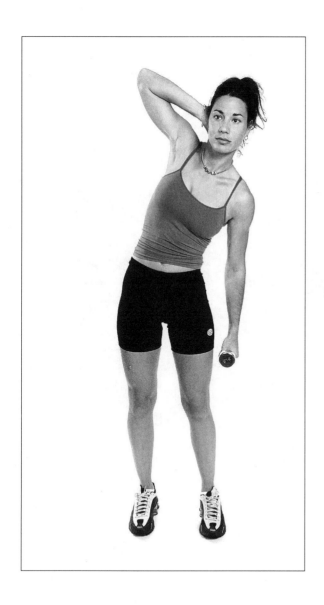

SIDE BENDS ON EXERCISE BALL

Place an exercise ball on the ground and lie sideways on the ball. The ball should be at your waist. Bend your bottom leg, kneeling on the ground, while extending your top leg. If you find it difficult to balance, brace your top foot against a wall. Place your hands behind your head, thumbs below your earlobes.

Leading with your top elbow, to the count of four, curl up sideways as far as you can go. Keep your head balanced and

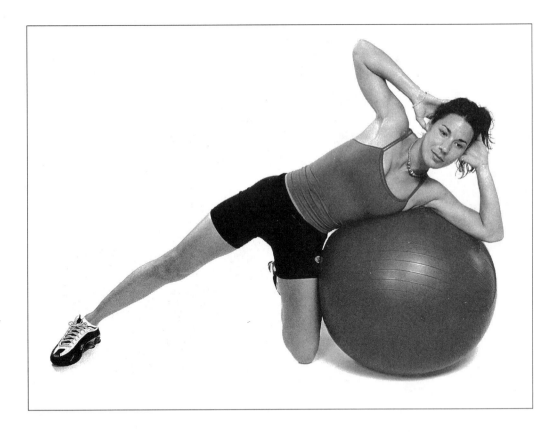

your back straight. Slowly return to the starting position to the count of four. After one set, switch sides.

12–15 repetitions • 2 sets each side

15–20 repetitions • 3 sets each side

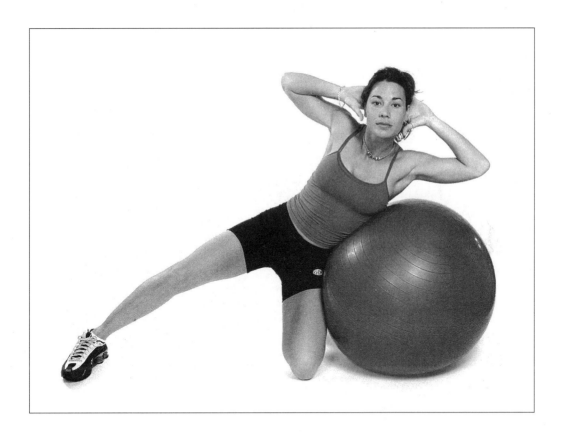

PART III

The Program

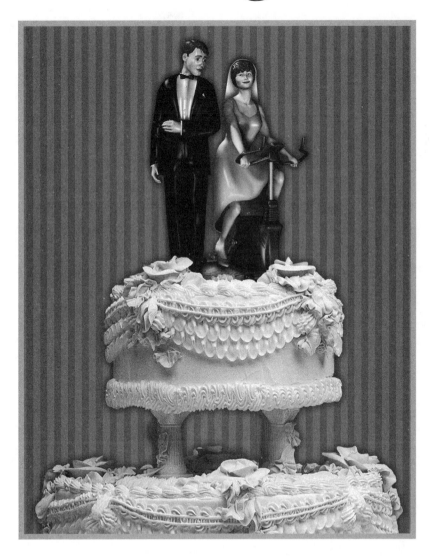

THE 24-WEEK STRENGTH TRAINING PROGRAM

have broken up the training program into 3 days a week for the first 12 weeks, then 4 days a week for the following 12 weeks. Feel free to change workout days; however, you should always give your muscles at least one day to recover between exercise sessions.

Note: Beginners can raise the intensity by doing two sets of each exercise.

- It is important to warm up by doing some light aerobic activity.

- Beginners should do only one set of each exercise during the first 2 weeks.

- Emphasize your form, take your time, and don't forget to breathe.

- For optimum results, a combination of flexibility, aerobic, and strength training is best.

- For easy reference, the page where each exercise can be found has been provided.

- I strongly recommend that you don't work out for 1 to 2 days before the big day.

Weeks 1-2

The following exercises will help you create a solid base. They have been designed to target the major muscle groups of the body. Do these for the first 2 weeks.

Monday, Wednesday, Friday

General
- Chest press, p. 56
- One-arm dumbbell rows, p. 52
- Dumbbell lunges, p. 34
- Alternating dumbbell curls, p. 72
- Dumbbell step-ups, p. 36
- Triceps kickbacks, p. 66
- Alternating front raises, p. 64
- Butt lifts with exercise ball, p. 44

Abdominals/Lower Back
- Raised-leg crunches on exercise ball, p. 80
- Superbrides, p. 54
- Dumbbell side bends, p. 82

Your cardiovascular workouts should be done during your off days, or they can be combined with your strength training routines. Your cardiovascular goal should be 60 to 80 minutes of aerobic activity in weeks 1 and 2. Pick one or more exercises that will enable you to elevate your heart rate and hold it for most of the workout. It is important that each aerobic session last at least 20 minutes. Refer to pages 17 to 22 for a more detailed discussion of cardiovascular exercise.

Refer to pages 17 to 22 for a more detailed discussion of cardiovascular exercise.

WEDDING TIP

*R*eserve photographer and/or videographer.

Weeks 3-4

Monday

General

Push-ups on exercise ball, p. 58

One-arm dumbbell rows, p. 52

Dumbbell lunges, p. 34

Alternating hammer curls, p. 74

Wall sits with exercise ball, p. 32

Triceps dips, p. 68

Lateral raises, p. 62

Bent-leg kickbacks, p. 48

Abdominals/Lower Back

Crunches on exercise ball, p. 78

Back extensions on exercise ball, p. 50

Side bends on exercise ball, p. 84

Wednesday

General

Chest press, p. 56

Seated overhead press, p. 60

Triceps extensions on exercise ball, p. 70

Wall sits with exercise ball, p. 32

Concentration biceps curls, p. 76

Bent-leg kickbacks, p. 48

Leg curls with exercise ball, p. 42

Lying adductions, p. 40

Abdominals/Lower Back

Raised-leg crunches on exercise ball, p. 80

Superbrides, p. 54

Side bends on exercise ball, p. 84

Friday

General

    Dumbbell step-ups, p. 36

    Push-ups on exercise ball, p. 58

    Wall sits with exercise ball, p. 32

    Triceps kickbacks, p. 66

    Alternating front raises, p. 64

    One-arm dumbbell rows, p. 52

    Lying bent-leg side raises, p. 38

    Butt lifts with exercise ball, p. 44

Abdominals/Lower Back

    Crunches on exercise ball, p. 78

    Back extensions on exercise ball, p. 50

    Dumbbell side bends, p. 82

 Your cardiovascular activity goal for weeks 3 to 4 should be 75 minutes per week. Pick one or more exercises that will enable you to elevate your heart rate and hold it for most of the workout. Each session should last at least 25 minutes.

WEDDING TIP

*B*egin to look at cakes and bakeries for the big day.

Weeks 5–6

Monday

General

Leg curls with exercise ball, p. 42

Chest press, p. 56

Lying adductions, p. 40

Standing kickbacks, p. 46

Lateral raises, p. 62

Triceps dips, p. 68

Alternating dumbbell curls, p. 72

Abdominals/Lower Back

Raised-leg crunches on exercise ball, p. 80

Superbrides, p. 54

Dumbbell side bends, p. 82

Wednesday

General

Dumbbell step-ups, p. 36

Bent-leg kickbacks, p. 48

Push-ups on exercise ball, p. 58

One-arm dumbbell rows, p. 52

Dumbbell lunges, p. 34

Alternating hammer curls, p. 74

Triceps extensions on exercise ball, p. 70

Lying bent-leg side raises, p. 38

Abdominals/Lower Back

Crunches on exercise ball, p. 78

Back extensions on exercise ball, p. 50

Side bends on exercise ball, p. 84

Friday

General

    Chest press, p. 56

    One-arm dumbbell rows, p. 52

    Wall sits with exercise ball, p. 32

    Alternating dumbbell curls, p. 72

    Dumbbell step-ups, p. 36

    Triceps kickbacks, p. 66

    Alternating front raises, p. 64

    Butt lifts with exercise ball, p. 44

Abdominals/Lower Back

    Raised-leg crunches on exercise ball, p. 84

    Superbrides, p. 54

    Dumbbell side bends, p. 82

Your cardiovascular activity goal for weeks 5 to 6 should be 75 to 80 minutes per week. Pick one or more exercises that will enable you to elevate your heart rate and hold it for most of the workout. Each session should last at least 25 minutes.

WEDDING TIP

*S*tart planning
your honeymoon.

Weeks 7-8

Monday
General

Push-ups on exercise ball, p. 58

One-arm dumbbell rows, p. 52

Dumbbell lunges, p. 34

Alternating hammer curls, p. 74

Wall sits with exercise ball, p. 32

Triceps dips, p. 68

Lateral raises, p. 62

Standing kickbacks, p. 46

Abdominals/Lower Back

Crunches on exercise ball, p. 78

Back extensions on exercise ball, p. 50

Side bends on exercise ball, p. 84

Wednesday
General

Chest press, p. 56

Seated overhead press, p. 60

Triceps extensions on exercise ball, p. 70

Wall sits with exercise ball, p. 32

Concentration biceps curls, p. 76

Butt lifts with exercise ball, p. 44

Leg curls with exercise ball, p. 42

Lying adductions, p. 40

Abdominals/Lower Back

Raised-leg crunches on exercise ball, p. 80

Superbrides, p. 54

Side bends on exercise ball, p. 84

Friday

General

    Dumbbell step-ups, p. 36

    Push-ups on exercise ball, p. 58

    Wall sits with exercise ball, p. 32

    Triceps kickbacks, p. 66

    Alternating front raises, p. 64

    One-arm dumbbell rows, p. 52

    Lying bent-leg side raises, p. 38

    Bent-leg kickbacks, p. 48

WEDDING TIP

*B*ook rehearsal-
dinner site.

Abdominals/Lower Back

    Crunches on exercise ball, p. 78

    Back extensions on exercise ball, p. 50

    Dumbbell side bends, p. 82

Your cardiovascular activity goal for weeks 7 to 8 should be 90 minutes per week. Pick one or more exercises that will enable you to elevate your heart rate and hold it for most of the workout. Each session should last at least 25 to 30 minutes.

Weeks **9–10**

Monday

General

Leg curls with exercise ball, p. 42

Chest press, p. 56

Lying adductions, p. 40

Standing kickbacks, p. 46

Lateral raises, p. 62

Triceps dips, p. 68

Alternating dumbbell curls, p. 72

Abdominals/Lower Back

Raised-leg crunches on exercise ball, p. 80

Superbrides, p. 54

Dumbbell side bends, p. 82

Wednesday

General

Dumbbell step-ups, p. 36

Bent-leg kickbacks, p. 48

Push-ups on exercise ball, p. 58

One-arm dumbbell rows, p. 52

Dumbbell lunges, p. 34

Alternating hammer curls, p. 74

Triceps extensions on exercise ball, p. 70

Seated overhead press, p. 60

Butt lifts with exercise ball, p. 44

Abdominals/Lower Back

Crunches on exercise ball, p. 78

Back extensions on exercise ball, p. 50

Side bends on exercise ball, p. 84

Friday

General

Chest press, p. 56

One-arm dumbbell rows, p. 52

Wall sits with exercise ball, p. 32

Alternating dumbbell curls, p. 72

Dumbbell step-ups, p. 36

Triceps kickbacks, p. 66

Alternating front raises, p. 64

Standing kickbacks, p. 46

WEDDING TIP

*D*ecide on a florist and floral scheme. Negotiate prices.

Abdominals/Lower Back

Raised-leg crunches on exercise ball, p. 80

Superbrides, p. 54

Dumbbell side bends, p. 82

Your cardiovascular activity goal for weeks 9 to 10 should be 90 to 105 minutes per week. Pick one or more exercises that will enable you to elevate your heart rate and hold it for most of the workout. Each session should last at least 30 to 35 minutes.

Weeks **11–12**

Monday

General

Dumbbell step-ups, p. 36

Chest press, p. 56

One-arm dumbbell rows, p. 52

Dumbbell lunges, p. 34

Alternating dumbbell curls, p. 72

Triceps kickbacks, p. 66

Alternating front raises, p. 64

Standing kickbacks, p. 46

Abdominals/Lower Back

Raised-leg crunches on exercise ball, p. 80

Superbrides, p. 54

Dumbbell side bends, p. 82

Wednesday

General

Push-ups on exercise ball, p. 58

Seated overhead press, p. 60

Triceps extensions on exercise ball, p. 70

Wall sits with exercise ball, p. 32

Concentration biceps curls, p. 76

Butt lifts with exercise ball, p. 44

Leg curls with exercise ball, p. 42

Abdominals/Lower Back

Raised-leg crunches on exercise ball, p. 80

Superbrides, p. 54

Side bends on exercise ball, p. 84

Friday

General

Dumbbell step-ups, p. 36

Chest press, p. 56

Bent-leg kickbacks, p. 48

Triceps kickbacks, p. 66

Alternating front raises, p. 64

One-arm dumbbell rows, p. 52

Lying bent-leg side raises, p. 38

Lying adductions, p. 40

Abdominals/Lower Back

Crunches on exercise ball, p. 78

Back extensions on exercise ball, p. 50

Dumbbell side bends, p. 82

WEDDING TIP

*P*ick up your invitations.

Your cardiovascular activity goal for weeks 11 to 12 should be 90 to 105 minutes per week. Pick one or more exercises that will enable you to elevate your heart rate and hold it for most of the workout. Each session should last at least 30 to 35 minutes.

Weeks 13–14

At this point in our 24-week program, add a fourth workout day to increase the intensity. The program will now incorporate more upper-body exercises for well-toned arms that will look fabulous in any gown!

Monday

General

One-arm dumbbell rows, p. 52

Alternating hammer curls, p. 74

Wall sits with exercise ball, p. 32

Triceps dips, p. 68

Lateral raises, p. 62

Standing kickbacks, p. 46

Concentration biceps curls, p. 76

Triceps extensions on exercise ball, p. 70

Abdominals/Lower Back

Crunches on exercise ball, p. 78

Back extensions on exercise ball, p. 50

Side bends on exercise ball, p. 84

Wednesday

General

Chest press, p. 56

Seated overhead press, p. 60

Triceps extensions on exercise ball, p. 70

Wall sits with exercise ball, p. 32

Concentration biceps curls, p. 76

Butt lifts with exercise ball, p. 44

Leg curls with exercise ball, p. 42

Alternating front raises, p. 64

Abdominals/Lower Back

Raised-leg crunches on exercise ball, p. 80

Superbrides, p. 54

Side bends on exercise ball, p. 84

Friday

General

Dumbbell step-ups, p. 36

Push-ups on exercise ball, p. 58

Alternating hammer curls, p. 74

Triceps kickbacks, p. 66

Alternating front raises, p. 64

One-arm dumbbell rows, p. 52

Lying bent-leg side raises, p. 38

Alternating dumbbell curls, p. 72

Abdominals/Lower Back

Crunches on exercise ball, p. 78

Back extensions on exercise ball, p. 50

Dumbbell side bends, p. 82

Saturday or Sunday

General

Chest press, p. 56

One-arm dumbbell rows, p. 52

Dumbbell lunges, p. 34

Alternating dumbbell curls, p. 72

Dumbbell step-ups, p. 36

Triceps kickbacks, p. 66

Alternating front raises, p. 64

Push-ups on exercise ball, p. 58

Bent-leg kickbacks, p. 48

Abdominals/Lower Back

Raised-leg crunches on exercise ball, p. 80

Superbrides, p. 54

Dumbbell side bends, p. 82

Your cardiovascular activity goal for weeks 13 to 14 should be 90 to 120 minutes per week. Pick one or more exercises that will enable you to elevate your heart rate and hold it for most of the workout. Each session should last at least 30 to 40 minutes.

WEDDING TIP

*C*onfirm the delivery date of your gown and schedule fittings.

Weeks **15–16**

Monday

General

Leg curls with exercise ball, p. 42

Chest press, p. 56

Lying adductions, p. 40

Standing kickbacks, p. 46

Lateral raises, p. 62

Alternating dumbbell curls, p. 72

Alternating front raises, p. 64

Triceps extensions on exercise ball, p. 70

Abdominals/Lower Back

Raised-leg crunches on exercise ball, p. 80

Superbrides, p. 54

Dumbbell side bends, p. 82

Wednesday

General

Dumbbell step-ups, p. 36

Bent-leg kickbacks, p. 48

Push-ups on exercise ball, p. 58

One-arm dumbbell rows, p. 52

Dumbbell lunges, p. 34

Alternating hammer curls, p. 74

Triceps extensions on exercise ball, p. 70

Concentration biceps curls, p. 76

Abdominals/Lower Back

Crunches on exercise ball, p. 78

Back extensions on exercise ball, p. 50

Side bends on exercise ball, p. 84

Friday

General

    Chest press, p. 56

    One-arm dumbbell rows, p. 52

    Wall sits with exercise ball, p. 32

    Alternating dumbbell curls, p. 72

    Dumbbell step-ups, p. 36

    Triceps kickbacks, p. 66

    Alternating front raises, p. 64

    Triceps extensions on exercise ball, p. 70

Abdominals/Lower Back

    Raised-leg crunches on exercise ball, p. 80

    Superbrides, p. 54

    Dumbbell side bends, p. 82

Saturday or Sunday

General

    Chest press, p. 56

    Push-ups on exercise ball, p. 58

    One-arm dumbbell rows, p. 52

    Dumbbell lunges, p. 34

    Alternating hammer curls, p. 74

    Wall sits with exercise ball, p. 32

    Triceps dips, p. 68

    Lateral raises, p. 62

    Butt lifts with exercise ball, p. 44

Abdominals/Lower Back

    Crunches on exercise ball, p. 78

    Back extensions on exercise ball, p. 50

    Side bends on exercise ball, p. 84

Your cardiovascular activity goal for weeks 15 to 16 should be 90 to 120 minutes per week. Pick one or more exercises that will enable you to elevate your heart rate and hold it for most of the workout. Each session should last at least 30 to 40 minutes.

Weeks **17–18**

Monday

General

One-arm dumbbell rows, p. 52

Butt lifts with exercise ball, p. 44

Alternating dumbbell curls, p. 72

Dumbbell step-ups, p. 36

Lateral raises, p. 62

Triceps kickbacks, p. 66

Alternating front raises, p. 64

Lying adductions, p. 40

Abdominals/Lower Back

Raised-leg crunches on exercise ball, p. 80

Superbrides, p. 54

Dumbbell side bends, p. 82

Wednesday

General

Push-ups on exercise ball, p. 58

One-arm dumbbell rows, p. 52

Dumbbell lunges, p. 34

Alternating dumbbell curls, p. 72

Wall sits with exercise ball, p. 32

Triceps dips, p. 68

Lateral raises, p. 62

Alternating hammer curls, p. 74

Abdominals/Lower Back

Crunches on exercise ball, p. 78

Back extensions on exercise ball, p. 50

Side bends on exercise ball, p. 84

Friday

General

Chest press, p. 56

Seated overhead press, p. 60

Triceps extensions on exercise ball, p. 70

Wall sits with exercise ball, p. 32

Concentration biceps curls, p. 76

Butt lifts with exercise ball, p. 44

Leg curls with exercise ball, p. 42

Triceps dips, p. 68

Abdominals/Lower Back

Raised-leg crunches on exercise ball, p. 80

Superbrides, p. 54

Side bends on exercise ball, p. 84

Saturday or Sunday

General

Chest press, p. 56

Dumbbell step-ups, p. 36

Push-ups on exercise ball, p. 58

Wall sits with exercise ball, p. 32

Triceps kickbacks, p. 66

Alternating front raises, p. 64

One-arm dumbbell rows, p. 52

Lying bent-leg side raises, p. 38

Abdominals/Lower Back

Crunches on exercise ball, p. 78

Back extensions on exercise ball, p. 50

Dumbbell side bends, p. 82

Your cardiovascular activity goal for weeks 17 to 18 should be 105 to 120 minutes per week. Pick one or more exercises that will enable you to elevate your heart rate and hold it for most of the workout. Each session should last at least 35 to 40 minutes.

Weeks 19–20

Monday
General

Leg curls with exercise ball, p. 42

Chest press, p. 56

Lying adductions, p. 40

Standing kickbacks, p. 46

Lateral raises, p. 62

Triceps dips, p. 68

Alternating dumbbell curls, p. 72

Alternating front raises, p. 64

Abdominals/Lower Back

Raised-leg crunches on exercise ball, p. 80

Superbrides, p. 54

Dumbbell side bends, p. 82

Wednesday
General

Dumbbell step-ups, p. 36

Bent-leg kickbacks, p. 48

Push-ups on exercise ball, p. 58

One-arm dumbbell rows, p. 52

Dumbbell lunges, p. 34

Alternating hammer curls, p. 74

Triceps extensions on exercise ball, p. 70

Concentration biceps curls, p. 76

Abdominals/Lower Back

Crunches on exercise ball, p. 78

Back extensions on exercise ball, p. 50

Side bends on exercise ball, p. 84

Friday

General

Chest press, p. 56

One-arm dumbbell rows, p. 52

Triceps dips, p. 68

Wall sits with exercise ball, p. 32

Alternating dumbbell curls, p. 72

Dumbbell step-ups, p. 36

Triceps kickbacks, p. 66

Alternating front raises, p. 64

Abdominals/Lower Back

Raised-leg crunches on exercise ball, p. 80

Superbrides, p. 54

Dumbbell side bends, p. 82

Saturday or Sunday

General

Chest press, p. 56

Push-ups on exercise ball, p. 58

One-arm dumbbell rows, p. 52

Dumbbell lunges, p. 34

Alternating hammer curls, p. 74

Wall sits with exercise ball, p. 32

Triceps dips, p. 68

Lateral raises, p. 62

Butt lifts with exercise ball, p. 44

Abdominals/Lower Back

Crunches on exercise ball, p. 78

Back extensions on exercise ball, p. 50

Side bends on exercise ball, p. 84

Your cardiovascular activity goal for weeks 19 to 20 should be 105 to 120 minutes per week. Pick one or more exercises that will enable you to elevate your heart rate and hold it for most of the workout. Each session should last at least 35 to 40 minutes.

Weeks 21–22

Monday
General

- Push-ups on exercise ball, p. 58
- One-arm dumbbell rows, p. 52
- Seated overhead press, p. 60
- Alternating hammer curls, p. 74
- Wall sits with exercise ball, p. 32
- Triceps dips, p. 68
- Lateral raises, p. 62
- Lying adductions, p. 40

Abdominals/Lower Back

- Crunches on exercise ball, p. 78
- Back extensions on exercise ball, p. 50
- Side bends on exercise ball, p. 84

Wednesday
General

- Leg curls with exercise ball, p. 42
- Chest press, p. 56
- Lying adductions, p. 40
- Alternating hammer curls, p. 74
- Standing kickbacks, p. 46
- Lateral raises, p. 62
- Triceps dips, p. 68
- Alternating dumbbell curls, p. 72

Abdominals/Lower Back

- Raised-leg crunches on exercise ball, p. 80
- Superbrides, p. 54
- Dumbbell side bends, p. 82

BUFF
Brides

Friday

General

Dumbbell step-ups, p. 36

Bent-leg kickbacks, p. 48

Push-ups on exercise ball, p. 58

One-arm dumbbell rows, p. 52

Alternating hammer curls, p. 74

Triceps extensions on exercise ball, p. 70

Lying bent-leg side raises, p. 38

Triceps dips, p. 68

Abdominals/Lower Back

Crunches on exercise ball, p. 78

Back extensions on exercise ball, p. 50

Side bends on exercise ball, p. 84

Saturday or Sunday

General

Chest press, p. 56

One-arm dumbbell rows, p. 52

Wall sits with exercise ball, p. 32

Alternating dumbbell curls, p. 72

Dumbbell step-ups, p. 36

Triceps kickbacks, p. 66

Alternating front raises, p. 64

Push-ups on exercise ball, p. 58

Butt lifts with exercise ball, p. 44

Abdominals/Lower Back

Raised-leg crunches on exercise ball, p. 80

Superbrides, p. 54

Dumbbell side bends, p. 82

Confirm date, location, time, and playlist with DJ or band.

Your cardiovascular activity goal for weeks 21 to 22 should be 120 minutes per week. Pick one or more exercises that will enable you to elevate your heart rate and hold it for most of the workout. Each session should last at least 40 minutes.

Weeks **23–24**

Monday

General

Chest press, p. 56

One-arm dumbbell rows, p. 52

Dumbbell lunges, p. 34

Lateral raises, p. 62

Alternating dumbbell curls, p. 72

Dumbbell step-ups, p. 36

Triceps kickbacks, p. 66

Alternating front raises, p. 64

Abdominals/Lower Back

Raised-leg crunches on exercise ball, p. 80

Superbrides, p. 54

Dumbbell side bends, p. 82

Wednesday

General

Chest press, p. 56

Seated overhead press, p. 60

Triceps extensions on exercise ball, p. 70

Wall sits with exercise ball, p. 32

Concentration biceps curls, p. 76

Butt lifts with exercise ball, p. 44

Leg curls with exercise ball, p. 42

Alternating dumbbell curls, p. 72

Abdominals/Lower Back

Raised-leg crunches on exercise ball, p. 80

Superbrides, p. 54

Side bends on exercise ball, p. 84

Friday

General

Dumbbell step-ups, p. 36

Push-ups on exercise ball, p. 58

Wall sits with exercise ball, p. 32

Triceps kickbacks, p. 66

Alternating front raises, p. 64

One-arm dumbbell rows, p. 52

Lying bent-leg side raises, p. 38

Triceps extensions on exercise ball, p. 70

Abdominals/Lower Back

Crunches on exercise ball, p. 78

Back extensions on exercise ball, p. 50

Dumbbell side bends, p. 82

Saturday or Sunday

General

Chest press, p. 56

One-arm dumbbell rows, p. 52

Dumbbell lunges, p. 34

Push-ups on exercise ball, p. 58

Alternating hammer curls, p. 74

Wall sits with exercise ball, p. 32

Triceps dips, p. 68

Lateral raises, p. 62

Standing kickbacks, p. 46

Abdominals/Lower Back

Crunches on exercise ball, p. 78

Back extensions on exercise ball, p. 50

Side bends on exercise ball, p. 84

WEDDING TIP

*C*onfirm big-day beauty appointments: for hair, nails, makeup.

❤ Your cardiovascular activity goal for weeks 22 to 24 should be 120 minutes per week. Pick one or more exercises that will enable you to elevate your heart rate and hold it for most of the workout. Each session should last at least 40 minutes.

Congratulations! You have completed the *Buff Brides* 24-week strength training program!

For brides-to-be who find themselves panicked three months before the wedding, this 12-week crash program is for you.

- Beginners should start with one set of each exercise for the first few sessions. If you experience only minimal soreness, you may move up to two sets of each exercise.

- I strongly recommend that you don't work out for 1 to 2 days before the big day.

Weeks 1–2

Monday

General

One-arm dumbbell rows, p. 52

Alternating hammer curls, p. 74

Wall sits with exercise ball, p. 32

Triceps dips, p. 68

Lateral raises, p. 62

Standing kickbacks, p. 46

Concentration biceps curls, p. 76

Triceps extensions on exercise ball, p. 70

Abdominals/Lower Back

Crunches on exercise ball, p. 78

Back extensions on exercise ball, p. 50

Side bends on exercise ball, p. 84

Wednesday

General

Chest press, p. 56

Seated overhead press, p. 60

Triceps extensions on exercise ball, p. 70

Wall sits with exercise ball, p. 32

Concentration biceps curls, p. 76

Butt lifts with exercise ball, p. 44

Leg curls with exercise ball, p. 42

Alternating front raises, p. 64

Abdominals/Lower Back

Raised-leg crunches on exercise ball, p. 80

Superbrides, p. 54

Side bends on exercise ball, p. 84

Friday

General

Dumbbell step-ups, p. 36

Push-ups on exercise ball, p. 58

Alternating hammer curls, p. 74

Triceps kickbacks, p. 66

Alternating front raises, p. 64

One-arm dumbbell rows, p. 52

Lying bent-leg side raises, p. 38
Alternating dumbbell curls, p. 72

Abdominals/Lower Back
Crunches on exercise ball, p. 78
Back extensions on exercise ball, p. 50
Dumbbell side bends, p. 82

Saturday or Sunday
General
Chest press, p. 56
One-arm dumbbell rows, p. 52
Dumbbell lunges, p. 34
Alternating dumbbell curls, p. 72
Dumbbell step-ups, p. 36
Triceps kickbacks, p. 66
Alternating front raises, p. 64
Push-ups on exercise ball, p. 58
Bent-leg kickbacks, p. 48

Abdominals/Lower Back
Raised-leg crunches on exercise ball, p. 80
Superbrides, p. 54
Dumbbell side bends, p. 82

WEDDING TIP

*C*onfirm the delivery
date of your gown and
schedule fittings.

Your cardiovascular activity goal for weeks 1 to 2 should be 60 minutes per week. Pick one or more exercises that will enable you to elevate your heart rate and hold it for most of the workout. Each session should last at least 20 minutes.

Weeks 3–4

Monday

General

Leg curls with exercise ball, p. 42

Chest press, p. 56

Lying adductions, p. 40

Standing kickbacks, p. 46

Lateral raises, p. 62

Alternating dumbbell curls, p. 72

Alternating front raises, p. 64

Triceps extensions on exercise ball, p. 70

Abdominals/Lower Back

Raised-leg crunches on exercise ball, p. 80

Superbrides, p. 54

Dumbbell side bends, p. 82

Wednesday

General

Dumbbell step-ups, p. 36

Bent-leg kickbacks, p. 48

Push-ups on exercise ball, p. 58

One-arm dumbbell rows, p. 52

Dumbbell lunges, p. 34

Alternating hammer curls, p. 74

Triceps extensions on exercise ball, p. 70

Concentration biceps curls, p. 76

Abdominals/Lower Back

Crunches on exercise ball, p. 78

Back extensions on exercise ball, p. 50

Side bends on exercise ball, p. 84

Friday

General

Chest press, p. 56

One-arm dumbbell rows, p. 52

Wall sits with exercise ball, p. 32

Alternating dumbbell curls, p. 72

Dumbbell step-ups, p. 36

Triceps kickbacks, p. 66

Alternating front raises, p. 64

Triceps extensions on exercise ball, p. 70

Abdominals/Lower Back

Raised-leg crunches on exercise ball, p. 80

Superbrides, p. 54

Dumbbell side bends, p. 82

Saturday or Sunday

General

Chest press, p. 56

Push-ups on exercise ball, p. 58

One-arm dumbbell rows, p. 52

Dumbbell lunges, p. 34

Alternating hammer curls, p. 74

Wall sits with exercise ball, p. 32

Triceps dips, p. 68

Lateral raises, p. 62

Butt lifts with exercise ball, p. 44

Abdominals/Lower Back

Crunches on exercise ball, p. 78

Back extensions on exercise ball, p. 50

Side bends on exercise ball, p. 84

Your cardiovascular activity goal for weeks 3 to 4 should be 60 to 75 minutes per week. Pick one or more exercises that will enable you to elevate your heart rate and hold it for most of the workout. Each session should last at least 20 to 25 minutes.

WEDDING TIP

*S*end out invitations.

Weeks **5–6**

Monday

General

One-arm dumbbell rows, p. 52

Butt lifts on exercise ball, p. 44

Alternating dumbbell curls, p. 72

Dumbbell step-ups, p. 36

Lateral raises, p. 62

Triceps kickbacks, p. 66

Alternating front raises, p. 64

Lying adductions, p. 40

Abdominals/Lower Back

Raised-leg crunches on exercise ball, p. 80

Superbrides, p. 54

Dumbbell side bends, p. 82

Wednesday

General

Push-ups on exercise ball, p. 58

One-arm dumbbell rows, p. 52

Dumbbell lunges, p. 34

Alternating dumbbell curls, p. 72

Wall sits with exercise ball, p. 32

Triceps dips, p. 68

Lateral raises, p. 62

Alternating hammer curls, p. 74

Abdominals/Lower Back

Crunches on exercise ball, p. 76

Back extensions on exercise ball, p. 50

Side bends on exercise ball, p. 84

Friday

General

Chest press, p. 56

Seated overhead press, p. 60

Triceps extensions on exercise ball, p. 70

Wall sits with exercise ball, p. 32

Concentration biceps curls, p. 76

Butt lifts with exercise ball, p. 44

Leg curls with exercise ball, p. 42

Triceps dips, p. 68

Abdominals/Lower Back

Raised-leg crunches on exercise ball, p. 80

Superbrides, p. 54

Side bends on exercise ball, p. 84

Saturday or Sunday

General

Chest press, p. 56

Dumbbell step-ups, p. 36

Push-ups on exercise ball, p. 58

Wall sits with exercise ball, p. 32

Triceps kickbacks, p. 66

Alternating front raises, p. 64

One-arm dumbbell rows, p. 52

Lying bent-leg side raises, p. 38

Abdominals/Lower Back

Crunches on exercise ball, p. 78

Back extensions on exercise ball, p. 50

Dumbbell side bends, p. 82

Your cardiovascular activity goal for weeks 5 to 6 should be 75 minutes per week. Pick one or more exercises that will enable you to elevate your heart rate and hold it for most of the workout. Each session should last at least 25 minutes.

Weeks **7–8**

Monday

General

Leg curls with exercise ball, p. 42

Chest press, p. 56

Lying adductions, p. 40

Standing kickbacks, p. 46

Lateral raises, p. 62

Triceps dips, p. 68

Alternating dumbbell curls, p. 72

Alternating front raises, p. 64

Abdominals/Lower Back

Raised-leg crunches on exercise ball, p. 80

Superbrides, p. 54

Dumbbell side bends, p. 82

Wednesday

General

Dumbbell step-ups, p. 36

Bent-leg kickbacks, p. 48

Push-ups on exercise ball, p. 58

One-arm dumbbell rows, p. 52

Dumbbell lunges, p. 34

Alternating hammer curls, p. 74

Triceps extensions on exercise ball, p. 70

Concentration biceps curls, p. 76

Abdominals/Lower Back

Crunches on exercise ball, p. 78

Back extensions on exercise ball, p. 50

Side bends on exercise ball, p. 84

Friday

General

Chest press, p. 56

One-arm dumbbell rows, p. 52

Triceps dips, p. 68

Wall sits with exercise ball, p. 32

Alternating dumbbell curls, p. 72

Dumbbell step-ups, p. 36

Triceps kickbacks, p. 66

Alternating front raises, p. 64

Abdominals/Lower Back

Raised-leg crunches on exercise ball, p. 80

Superbrides, p. 54

Dumbbell side bends, p. 82

Saturday or Sunday

General

Push-ups on exercise ball, p. 58

One-arm dumbbell rows, p. 52

Dumbbell lunges, p. 34

Alternating hammer curls, p. 74

Wall sits with exercise ball, p. 32

Triceps dips, p. 68

Lateral raises, p. 62

Chest press, p. 56

Butt lifts with exercise ball, p. 44

Abdominals/Lower Back

Crunches on exercise ball, p. 78

Back extensions on exercise ball, p. 50

Side bends on exercise ball, p. 84

BUFF
Brides

Your cardiovascular activity goal for weeks 7 to 8 should be 75 to 90 minutes per week. Pick one or more exercises that will enable you to elevate your heart rate and hold it for most of the workout. Each session should last at least 25 to 30 minutes.

WEDDING TIP

Put together the seating chart for the reception. Make place cards.

Weeks **9–10**

Monday

General

Push-ups on exercise ball, p. 58

One-arm dumbbell rows, p. 52

Seated overhead press, p. 60

Alternating hammer curls, p. 74

Wall sits with exercise ball, p. 32

Triceps dips, p. 68

Lateral raises, p. 62

Lying adductions, p. 40

Abdominals/Lower Back

Crunches on exercise ball, p. 78

Back extensions on exercise ball, p. 50

Side bends on exercise ball, p. 84

Wednesday

General

Leg curls with exercise ball, p. 42

Chest press, p. 56

Lying adductions, p. 40

Alternating hammer curls, p. 74

Standing kickbacks, p. 46

Lateral raises, p. 62

Triceps dips, p. 68

Alternating dumbbell curls, p. 72

Abdominals/Lower Back

Raised-leg crunches on exercise ball, p. 80

Superbrides, p. 54

Dumbbell side bends, p. 82

Friday

General

Dumbbell step-ups, p. 36

Bent-leg kickbacks, p. 48

Push-ups on exercise ball, p. 58

One-arm dumbbell rows, p. 52

Alternating hammer curls, p. 74

Triceps extensions on exercise ball, p. 70

Lying bent-leg side raises, p. 38

Triceps dips, p. 68

Abdominals/Lower Back

Crunches on exercise ball, p. 78

Back extensions on exercise ball, p. 50

Side bends on exercise ball, p. 84

Saturday or Sunday

General

Chest press, p. 56

One-arm dumbbell rows, p. 52

Wall sits with exercise ball, p. 32

Alternating dumbbell curls, p. 72

Dumbbell step-ups, p. 36

Triceps kickbacks, p. 66

Alternating front raises, p. 64

Push-ups on exercise ball, p. 58

Butt lifts on exercise ball, p. 44

Your cardiovascular activity goal for weeks 9 to 10 should be 90 minutes per week. Pick one or more exercises that will enable you to elevate your heart rate and hold it for most of the workout. Each session should last at least 30 minutes.

WEDDING TIP

*C*onfirm date, location, time, and playlist with DJ or band.

Weeks **11–12**

Monday

General

 Chest press, p. 56

 One-arm dumbbell rows, p. 52

 Dumbbell lunges, p. 34

 Lateral raises, p. 62

 Alternating dumbbell curls, p. 72

 Dumbbell step-ups, p. 36

 Triceps kickbacks, p. 66

 Alternating front raises, p. 64

Abdominals/Lower Back

 Raised-leg crunches on exercise ball, p. 80

 Superbrides, p. 54

 Dumbbell side bends, p. 82

Wednesday

General

 Chest press, p. 56

 Seated overhead press, p. 60

 Triceps extensions on exercise ball, p. 70

 Wall sits with exercise ball, p. 32

 Concentration biceps curls, p. 76

 Butt lifts with exercise ball, p. 44

 Leg curls with exercise ball, p. 42

 Alternating dumbbell curls, p. 72

Abdominals/Lower Back

 Raised-leg crunches on exercise ball, p. 80

 Superbrides, p. 54

 Side bends on exercise ball, p. 84

Friday

General

Dumbbell step-ups, p. 36

Push-ups on exercise ball, p. 58

Wall sits with exercise ball, p. 32

Triceps kickbacks, p. 66

Alternating front raises, p. 64

One-arm dumbbell rows, p. 52

Lying bent-leg side raises, p. 38

Triceps extensions on exercise ball, p. 70

Abdominals/Lower Back

Crunches on exercise ball, p. 78

Back extensions on exercise ball, p. 50

Dumbbell side bends, p. 82

Saturday or Sunday

General

Chest press, p. 56

One-arm dumbbell rows, p. 52

Dumbbell lunges, p. 34

Push-ups on exercise ball, p. 58

Alternating hammer curls, p. 74

Wall sits with exercise ball, p. 32

Triceps dips, p. 68

Lateral raises, p. 62

Standing kickbacks, p. 46

Abdominals/Lower Back

Crunches on exercise ball, p. 78

Back extensions on exercise ball, p. 50

Side bends on exercise ball, p. 84

Your cardiovascular activity goal for weeks 11 to 12 should be 105 minutes per week. Pick one or more exercises that will enable you to elevate your heart rate and hold it for most of the workout. Each session should last at least 35 minutes.

Congratulations! You have completed the *Buff Brides* 12-week crash program!

ACKNOWLEDGMENTS

Although there is only one name on the cover, every book is a collaborative effort and that holds true for this one.

My sincere thanks to Ivan Held at Random House for his invaluable support. His belief in this project from the beginning enabled it to finally get off the ground. Also, thank you to Gretchen Koss, my dear friend, who was instrumental in making this all happen; thanks to Molly Stern and Tracy Locke for their expertise and advice.

Special thanks to my editor, Janelle Duryea; your enthusiasm, help, and guidance were irreplaceable. Thanks to the support of Bruce Tracy, Dan Rembert, Jynne Martin, and all the hardworking people at Villard.

I would like to thank jacket designer and illustrator Jack Myers and interior photographer Lisa Graziano. The creativity and passion the two of you put into this project make this book one of a kind.

Thanks to Karen Shatzkin for your astute legal advice; stylist and friend April Troiani; dear friends and clients Allison and David Rich; interior model Alycia Kluegl; the professional advice of trainer Monica Ward; Libby Clark and New York Sports Club; and Kate Niedzwiecki.

Thank you to my friends and colleagues at the Riverdale Country School for your constant support.

I also want to extend my deepest gratitude and affection to the following people. Because of your love, friendship, and endless support, this book is as much for you as it is for me: Lauren Van Kirk, Suzanne Borda, Polly Defrank, Bonnie Eldon, Sandra DeOvando, Deborah Larkin, Kenny Goldblatt, Kelly Donlon, Donna Bugdin, Jackie Bertone, Dina DiMaria, Matthew Robbins, Jen Abbondanza, Alan Slater, Karen Vetrone, and Honor MacNaughton.

ACKNOWLEDGMENTS

INDEX

Q

quadriceps exercises, 31–37
  dumbbell lunges, 34–35
  dumbbell step-ups, 36–37
  wall sits with exercise ball, 32–33
quadriceps muscles, description
    of, 31
quadriceps stretches, 11
questions commonly asked, xiii–xv

R

repetitions, of exercises, xiv, 23
resting, between exercises, xv
running, 19–20
running shoes, 19–20

S

"saddle-bags," 38
seated overhead press, 60–61
self-motivation, 3–4
sets, of exercises, 23, 89, 118
shoes:
  running, 19–20
  walking, 19
shoulder exercises, 60–65
  alternating front raises, 64–65
  lateral raises, 62–63
  seated overhead press, 60–61
shoulders/middle of upper back
    stretches, 15
side bends, 82–85
  with dumbbells, 82–83, 90
  on exercise ball, 84–85
six-month program, xiii, 89–117
  weeks 1–2, 90
  weeks 3–4, 91–92
  weeks 5–6, 93–94
  weeks 7–8, 95–96
  weeks 9–10, 97–98
  weeks 11–12, 99–100

weeks 13–14, 101–3
weeks 15–16, 104–6
weeks 17–18, 107–8
weeks 19–20, 109–11
weeks 21–22, 112–14
weeks 23–24, 115–17
slim brides, 26, 27
soreness, muscular, xv, 5
spot reduction, xiv
standing kickbacks, 46–47
steps (benches), 8–9, 10
steps, exercises with:
  chest press, 56–57
  dumbbell step-ups, 36–37
  one-arm dumbbell rows,
    52–53
  seated overhead press, 60–61
  triceps dips, 68–69
  triceps kickbacks, 66–67
strength training, x, 5, 17,
    22–24
  importance of, 23
  soreness and, xv
  tips on, 23–24
  weights and repetitions and, xiv
stretches, xv, 5, 10–15, 17, 23
  butt, 13
  calf, 12
  chest/shoulder, 14
  groin, 15
  hamstring, 12
  importance of, 10, 20
  lower back/hip/hamstring, 13
  quadriceps, 11
  shoulders/middle of upper
    back, 15
  tips for, 10–11
  triceps, 14
superbrides, 54–55
supinating, 20

ABOUT THE AUTHOR

S U E   F L E M I N G earned her B.S. and M.S. in physical education and has been a certified personal trainer for the past ten years. She is currently the director of physical education at Riverdale Country School in Riverdale, New York, and continues to work with private clients, many of whom are brides-to-be. Fleming lives in Manhattan.